Riding the Lightning

RIDING
THE
LIGHTNING

A Year in the Life of a
New York City Paramedic

ANTHONY ALMOJERA

MARINER BOOKS
Boston   New York

RIDING THE LIGHTNING. Copyright © 2022 by Anthony Almojera. All rights reserved. Printed in the United States of America. No part of this book may be used or reproduced in any manner whatsoever without written permission except in the case of brief quotations embodied in critical articles and reviews. For information, address HarperCollins Publishers, 195 Broadway, New York, NY 10007.

HarperCollins books may be purchased for educational, business, or sales promotional use. For information, please email the Special Markets Department at SPsales@harpercollins.com.

FIRST EDITION

Designed by Chloe Foster

Library of Congress Cataloging-in-Publication Data has been applied for.
ISBN 978-0-358-65290-8

22 23 24 25 26 LSC 10 9 8 7 6 5 4 3 2 1

To broken people everywhere

Contents

Author's Note

The story that follows represents my views and not those of the Fire Department of the City of New York or its emergency medical services. It is based on interviews and other research as well as my own records and recollection. Out of respect for people's privacy, I have changed the names and identifying details of certain patients. Otherwise, the people, places, events, and dialogue described in the book are accurate to the best of my knowledge. Any errors are mine alone.

Prologue

Very early one Sunday in March 2020, I parked my crimson EMS truck outside a brick house in Sheepshead Bay. The neighborhood is on the southern edge of Brooklyn, right by the ocean. When I was a kid, it was full of Russian and Jewish families, but now there are people from all over—former Soviet states, Asia. It's a cultural mishmash. During normal times, after a call in this neighborhood I'd swing by Randazzo's Clam Bar and pick up a cup of chowder.

But these were not normal times.

An ambulance had reached the scene first and stopped just outside the house. Two paramedics were climbing out. I put on a gown and gloves and a surgical mask and followed the medics—also gowned and masked—around the side of the house to an apartment on the ground floor. The front door had been left ajar, which is what 911 dispatchers tell callers to do. We stepped inside.

A woman lay unconscious on the floor of the living room. She was petite and had straight dark hair and she wore a white blouse or night-gown of some sort. She looked like she was from the Philippines, like my grandfather.

A man was kneeling beside her. He also looked Filipino. He wore green scrubs. He had a slight build, but he was pumping the woman's chest with precise, strong movements. Most nonmedical people don't compress the chest as deeply as necessary when they perform CPR.

It's hard to do, and it can be brutal; you have to push with so much force that you can crack the sternum. But this guy clearly knew what he was doing.

The crew got down on the floor and took over CPR. The guy stood up and turned to me. The woman was his wife, he said. She had been sick for about five days. She'd been spiking fevers and coughing, and her chest hurt. The couple had not been tested for COVID-19, the man said, but the woman worked at a nursing home in Coney Island, so he figured she probably had the virus. I agreed.

The husband told me that he worked at a nearby hospital. He had stayed home for the past few days to look after his wife. But the night before, the hospital had called. "They were slammed," the guy said. "They begged me to come in. I didn't want to leave her. But she said that she would be okay. She told me not to worry about her, that I should go to work."

He held his palm to his forehead and closed his eyes.

"When I got home, she wasn't breathing," he said.

By then, an emergency medical technician crew had arrived. The EMTs were helping the paramedics from the first ambulance work up the patient (that is, perform CPR and give medications). There wasn't a lot of space in the room, so the husband stepped outside.

One of the paramedics put a bag-valve mask—a device for ventilating an unconscious patient—over the patient's nose and mouth. Her partner placed three electrode pads, white pads with colored cables, on the patient's chest so we could get a three-lead EKG. The cables were connected to a defibrillator with a cardiac monitor that showed the heart rhythm.

The woman's heart was in asystole—meaning there was no heartbeat, no indication of electrical activity.

We started an IV and gave the patient an amp of epinephrine, which increases blood flow to vital organs. All the while, we continued CPR. The woman had been unconscious and possibly not breathing for at least twenty minutes before we arrived. But we wanted to keep blood flowing through her body in case there was a chance that she could be saved.

I called telemetry—online medical control—to discuss medication with the physician on duty. Telemetry physicians help direct emergency medical care in the field. They authorize the use of certain medications and make the call on when to pronounce a patient dead.

The physician ordered doses of sodium bicarbonate and calcium chloride. Sodium bicarbonate lowers the acidity of the blood, which often rises during cardiac arrest, and calcium can help the heart beat more forcefully. We normally administer these drugs only when epinephrine and CPR aren't working. If the patient doesn't respond to these medications, there's nothing more we can do.

We continued CPR for ten minutes or so. We stopped every two minutes to check the patient's heart rhythm and have a new person take over CPR so no one became too tired to do it properly. We were looking for electrical activity on the monitor. Even better, a pulse—a sign that the heart had begun to pump again.

But there was nothing.

We worked on the patient for half an hour. Maybe fifty minutes had passed since her husband had found her unconscious. She wasn't responding to treatment. We were not going to save her.

I called telemetry again, this time to get permission to pronounce her. The physician gave me a time of death.

I stepped outside. The husband was pacing on the driveway next to a small sedan. My mouth felt dry. He had been forced to choose between caring for strangers and staying home to nurse the person he loved most in the world. He had gone to work, and his wife had died alone.

Could he have saved her if he had been home? Perhaps. A patient who receives CPR immediately after collapsing has a far better chance of survival than someone who doesn't, even if the delay is just a few minutes. If the husband had been home, he'd have been able to keep his wife's blood flowing while he waited for us to arrive. That might have been enough. Might not have. He'd never know.

The man and his wife could have been any of us, I thought—any of the emergency medical technicians and paramedics and nurses and doctors who were risking infection from the coronavirus every day. Any of us could wind up dead on the living-room floor. For my part, I live alone. If I got COVID and my heart gave out in the middle of the night, it could be hours before somebody found me.

I stopped on the edge of the grass, maybe eight feet from the man and his car. Under normal circumstances, I would have walked over to him to break the news quietly. I would have placed my hand on his forearm or his shoulder. But it was highly probable that he was infected. So I kept my distance.

The guy stopped pacing and turned toward me.

"I'm very sorry," I said. My voice was muffled by the mask. I cleared my throat. "I'm sorry," I said more loudly. "We've done everything we can. We gave her the same medications that she would have received in the hospital," I continued. "We used the same procedures. But she's in asystole."

The man worked in medicine, so he knew what this meant: his wife's heart wasn't responding. She had flatlined.

"There's nothing more we can do," I said.

The man's eyes widened. I saw his knees buckle. "No!" he yelled. "No, no, no." He put his fist to his mouth.

I felt an urge to cross the grass and put my arm around him. We hadn't been able to save his wife; the least I could do was console him. But I had to stay clear. So I just stood there in my stupid yellow gown and my purple gloves with my mask covering my face. "I'm sorry," I repeated.

The man turned and pounded the roof of his car. He kicked the fender. He kicked it again. He attacked the car as if he were trying to beat the life out of it. And then he melted to the ground, shoulders heaving.

The paramedics came out of the house, leaving the second crew inside to stay with the patient's body until the cops came. These paramedics were from Lutheran—officially NYU Langone Hospital–Brooklyn, but the facility used to be NYU Lutheran Medical Center and that name stuck. I knew one of them from my early days in emergency medicine, but this wasn't a moment for chitchat.

We stood in silence, looking at the crumpled man. Then I turned and walked back to my EMS truck. I climbed into the driver's seat. I tore off my mask. And tears wet my cheeks.

For nearly two decades, I have been a medical responder with the Fire Department of the City of New York's emergency medical services. The FDNY runs the bulk of ambulances in New York City. I've witnessed stillbirths, abused children, dismembered bodies, suicides. But before coronavirus hit New York, in the spring of 2020, I had never cried on the job.

The pandemic was like nothing I had ever experienced. It crashed into New York like a hurricane. It caught the city off guard—residents, government officials, hospital staff, schoolteachers. Everyone. Between mid-March and late April, COVID-19 killed somewhere between seventeen thousand and twenty-one thousand New Yorkers. That's many times more people than were killed in the attacks on the World Trade Center on September 11, 2001. EMS workers witnessed death after death—whole households falling sick, people dying because they couldn't afford to skip a supermarket shift. We weren't saving anyone, and we couldn't even comfort those left behind, all the countless bereaved New Yorkers, like the desperate man in Sheepshead Bay.

The pandemic broke us. After the disaster of the spring, a wave of grief and anxiety hit members of the emergency medical services. Some EMS members killed themselves. Some headed for the door.

Many who were close to retirement quit. They had worked the World Trade Center attacks two decades prior, and now they had worked through weeks of mayhem as the virus devoured New York. They had finally had enough.

But the truth is, the FDNY's emergency medical service—one of the largest and busiest in the United States—was broken before anyone had even heard of COVID-19. Our members were underpaid. Our infrastructure was aging and poorly organized. Our chiefs were out of touch. EMS was a rickety house with a leaky roof and rotten floorboards. A tropical storm could have blown it over, and we were hit by a category 5 hurricane. We didn't stand a chance.

Going into the pandemic, EMS wasn't the service that New York City deserved. Very few members stayed for more than five years. They couldn't make a living, and the benefits were poor. So it had become a corps of novices. At the height of the coronavirus crisis, I had emergency medical technicians with six months' experience running an ambulance with kids who were fresh out of the academy. They coped incredibly well. But it wasn't fair to them. And it's not how you run a world-class emergency medical service.

I didn't weather the pandemic so well myself. I'd thought I could handle anything my job threw at me. That I could witness any amount of suffering. That I was someone people could lean on. After all, I was the senior paramedic, the man who could restart a person's heart or detect a ruptured aneurysm and save a guy from bleeding to death internally; I was the union vice president, the one who blasted the higher-ups on Twitter and butted heads with them in person to defend my coworkers' rights. I was also the guy who cooked a nine-course meal for his friends at Christmas and organized group vacations to Hong Kong and Dublin and Uganda. I thought that I had all the answers.

But when the virus hit, I was feeling drained and disillusioned. I was worn out by my job and the frustrations of fighting for better pay and benefits. I had a work-related injury that meant I couldn't carry anything heavy in a job where lifting deadweight was routine. I had lost my parents—not that they were easy to deal with when they were alive. I'd lost my brother and had fallen out of touch with my sister. On top of that, I was in a relationship that was unraveling. I was about to be single yet again.

It wasn't just the FDNY's EMS—I was pretty unsteady too.

Riding the Lightning

OCTOBER 2019

It was after Joe Cengiz fell sick that things really started to go badly. That was before Wuhan locked down and before the hospitals in Northern Italy filled up. Before there were runs on toilet paper and N95 masks. Before they built a hospital in Central Park. For me, it began with Joe collapsing on the floor of his dining room in his underwear. That call marked the start of a year that turned out to be one of the hardest of my life.

When I walked into the dining room that October morning, Joe was leaning back against a leg of the big polished table in the center. The table was the color of maple syrup, and it filled the room and left little space for us to move. It didn't help that there were so many of us—cops, firefighters, emergency medical technicians, paramedics, Joe's brother-in-law Dino. Joe's sister Serpil was in the hallway outside. She couldn't get to her brother because there were so many people squeezed around that big table.

The only other piece of furniture I remember was a china closet. It was filled with plates, white and deep-sea blue.

Sweat ran down Joe's neck and formed rivulets between the white hairs on his chest. He had been in the shower, and his skin was still wet. The water mingled with heavy sweat oozing from his pores. Something was very wrong.

Diaphoresis—profuse sweating—is a classic symptom of an MI, a myocardial infarction. Heart attack, in other words. When there's a disruption to your circulation, your body sends all the blood to the vital organs and stops sending it to the periphery. You get dizzy. You sweat.

I saw a medic kneeling beside Joe. She talked to him softly. I recognized her. Sharon. She had worked with Joe at Station 38. Sharon had the cardiac monitor set up to check his heart, and she was wiping the sweat from his chest with tissues so that she could stick electrodes to his skin. Sharon was an experienced medic, but her hands shook as she tried to stick on the pads. It's one thing to treat a stranger; it's another to treat family. And to us, Joe was family.

I also knew Joe's literal family, a fact that ratcheted up the pressure even more. I had hung out with Serpil and Dino. I knew how close they were to Joe. They lived in the building next door and talked about living under one roof when they grew old. And they had been Joe's first call; he'd dialed Serpil and Dino when he realized something was wrong. Dino happened to be closest, and he'd reached Joe first. Now Dino stood at the other end of the dining table, looking extremely nervous.

I crouched in front of Joe. "Hey," I said. "What's going on?"

Joe raised his head. His skin was normally copper-colored and weathered, like a fisherman's. Now it was a sickly gray.

His face filled with relief. "Anthony," Joe said. "Thank God you're here."

When Joe keeled over with his chest on fire, I was wrists-deep in a bowl of raw meat. I'm a lieutenant paramedic at the Fire Department of New York's emergency medical services Station 40 in Sunset Park in Brooklyn. It was late October, a Saturday, and I was working a double shift, six a.m. to ten p.m.

Saturday mornings can be quiet, so I try to cook for the ambulance crews. Today I was prepping what would be a late lunch: meat loaf the way my mom used to make it—with pork, beef chuck, and veal.

Meat loaf was one of the few things my mom cooked well. Medics spend hours every day parked on street corners in the ambulance or driving between hospitals and patients' homes, so they eat a lot of crap. Cooking is a way to get everyone to sit together for a while and eat real food. It helps the ambulance crews bond. And we have a good kitchen at the station—stainless-steel counters, a stove with six burners, cooking pots like oil drums.

I was mixing the ingredients when my cell phone rang. For a second, I thought it might be the woman I was dating. She was mainly a texter, but every time my phone rang, I hoped it was her. I rinsed my hands.

"Anthony?" Not my girlfriend. It was Taisha Robinson, a lieutenant at Station 58 in Canarsie in Southeast Brooklyn. "We have an MOS who needs help," she said. *MOS* is shorthand for *member of service*—one of our brothers or sisters in EMS. "Heart problem, difficulty breathing. Bensonhurst," Taisha said. "I don't have a name."

As a lieutenant paramedic, I supervise ambulance crews that respond to 911 calls in New York City, specifically in Brooklyn South. Every FDNY ambulance is staffed with a pair of emergency medical technicians or paramedics. Outsiders might not be able to tell EMTs and paramedics apart, but there are differences, and they're significant.

Emergency medical technicians perform basic life support (BLS). They can give you oxygen if you're short of breath or glucose if you're hypoglycemic. They can pump your chest and pack a gunshot wound. They can save your life in myriad ways. But there is a limit to what EMTs are allowed to do. They can't give many medications, they can't start IVs, and they can't interpret a twelve-lead electrocardiogram, which gives a complex picture of the heart's electrical activity. That's the work of paramedics.

Paramedics have usually put in a few years as EMTs and spent hundreds of hours in paramedic school. They provide advanced life support (ALS). They can administer at least thirty-five medications;

they can drill a needle into a patient's tibia to administer fluids or medication. Their ambulance—or "bus," as it's known to EMS workers—is a mini–emergency room on wheels.

And then there are the lieutenant paramedics—like me—also known as "conditions bosses," because when they arrive on scene, they're in charge of the situation, or "conditions." As a lieutenant, I drive a conditions unit or command vehicle, a Chevy Silverado that most of us call simply "the truck." I'm assigned to complex emergencies—cardiac arrests, major injuries, fires—where the ambulance crews need support from a senior medic. If you cut your finger, I'm probably not going to supervise the call. If you stop breathing, I'll be there. I make sure the crews are handling things right. If necessary, I step in or organize additional backup.

When an MOS needs an ambulance, a lieutenant paramedic always joins the crew on the call. Always. Taisha called me directly because she knew I was in the area, and she wanted to speed things up.

The two-way radio that was propped on the kitchen counter crackled. The dispatcher's voice came over: "Five-Eight Zebra, take it to eighty-six hundred Bay Parkway for the sick MOS." Which meant Fifty-Eight Zebra, an ambulance from Taisha's station, was being dispatched to help a member of service. I jumped on the radio.

"Put me on the back of Five-Eight Zebra," I said. *Assign me to the call so I can support that ambulance crew.* I stashed the meat in the fridge and headed out.

Station 40 is a twenty-minute drive from Bay Parkway and Eighty-Sixth Street. The speed limit in New York is twenty-five miles an hour, and they say that traffic nowadays moves at about the same pace as a horse and cart. But if you go lights and sirens, you can do fifty miles an hour on the avenues, sixty or seventy on the expressways. I figured I'd make it in ten minutes.

I flew south on Seventh Avenue through Brooklyn's Chinatown, passing the grocers and the nail salons and the gastroenterologist and the dry cleaner where the medics at the station drop their uniforms. I hit the big dip on Sixty-Second that I always try to avoid; it sent the truck flying. I hung a left on Sixty-Fifth Street by the blue-and-white-painted Swedish Football Club that's left over from the days when the neighborhood was Scandinavian. Went past the Dust Bowl, where I'd played football as a kid, and past the corner where there used to be a muffler shop that my brother, Richie, worked at between his stints in jail.

As I drove, I tried to figure out who the patient might be. I've been in EMS for eighteen years and I've worked at most of the stations in the city. Even though I'm based in Brooklyn, I pick up overtime all over town—the Bronx, Harlem, Queens. On top of that, I'm vice president of the Uniformed EMS Officers Union Local 3621. I represent the senior EMS ranks. In short, I have a lot of contact with service members, so I figured it was very possible that I knew the MOS we were racing to help.

I swung right onto Eighteenth Avenue in Bensonhurst, shot past the gelato line at Villabate Alba and the Italian pork stores. Bensonhurst used to be pure Italian. A lot of mobsters. I grew up in Park Slope, five miles north and a world away, albeit in the days before Park Slope was full of progressives who would drop $3 million for a brownstone. When I was a teenager, a friend of my brother offered me a hundred dollars a run to carry packages from our neighborhood to Bensonhurst. Every day for a few weeks, I rode the bus to a social club on Eighteenth Avenue and handed a padded envelope to a guy named Dominic. I knew better than to look inside.

I headed east on Eighty-Sixth Street, going under the steel girders of the elevated D train. I pushed past oncoming traffic, forcing the cars to pull aside, then made a right on Bay Parkway.

And that's when it hit me. I recognized these buildings—1930s brick with fire escapes that were painted a rusty red. I pulled up behind the ambulance.

Shit, I thought. *It's Joe.*

• • •

Cemal Cengiz was a recently retired lieutenant EMT who'd spent fourteen years at Station 38, bang next door to Kings County Hospital in East Flatbush. (In those days, EMTs could be promoted to lieutenants; nowadays, only paramedics can.) I had worked at that station with Joe for seven years. A Crimean Turk, he had a bulbous nose, big brown eyes, and a white mustache shaped like the head of a push broom. The *C*s in his name were pronounced like *J*s. He called himself Joe.

Joe became Java Joe on account of the fact that he always carried a cup of coffee. Auditing the ALS equipment at the station, checking time sheets, driving the command vehicle—he was never without his coffee. Given the choice, he'd drink Turkish espresso with cardamom, but normally it was just a cup of brew from Dunkin' Donuts.

Joe had come to New York when he was a kid. His brother, Fazil, bought a couple of taxi medallions, and when Joe was older, Fazil told him to drive one of the taxis. Joe hated it. In the 1970s, Fazil also bought a dance studio in a big building near Times Square. It was a legendary place. Everyone went there to teach and rehearse. During the holidays, Joe's family would doll up the building and put up a big tree and throw a party.

I joined Station 38 in 2005, just after I'd qualified as a paramedic. I'd been an emergency medical technician for a couple of years and then gone to paramedic school, and now I was full of piss and vinegar. Ready to save the world with my new skills. But Joe just put his hands up and said, "Take it easy, Anthony. You'll see. This is a long career."

Joe was my kind of lieutenant. He let you do your job. If you screwed up, he didn't yell or embarrass you in front of people; he talked to you quietly afterward. Joe didn't push the departmental orthodoxy either. He knew that if you always followed the rules to the letter, it would take three hours to treat every patient, so he showed us the gray area that we needed to stay in in order to last in this profession.

One time, my ambulance pulled up at an apartment building on Empire Boulevard to treat a woman who had hurt her arm. Joe was the lieutenant assigned to the call. I took out the stair chair—a metal frame that makes it easier to transport patients up and down steps—so we could carry the patient out of the building. That was the rule: you carried the patient from the scene of the emergency to the ambulance.

"What are you doing with that?" Joe said. "You gonna carry every patient for twenty-five years? Save your back," he said. "She can walk."

Joe was all about doing the job without killing yourself.

Outside Station 38 there was a tree with a patch of dirt around it. Joe planted sunflowers there. The station was on a bare block, kind of ugly, with the hospital behind it and the medical examiner's office opposite. But Joe had these tall sunflowers with their golden heads growing out of a little bit of dust. He was so proud of them. After he got the station set up in the morning, he would get the dustpan and brush and he'd go out front and sweep. Then he would sit outside on a foldout chair with his coffee in his hand and chat with everyone. It was like he brought a little bit of Turkey with him.

As the years wore on, Joe became fixated on retirement. He planned to return to Turkey. He bought a plot of land there, near the coastal city of Izmir. He would build a house on the land, he said, and open a coffee shop. There was just one catch: he needed to work until he was sixty-two in order to retire on full pay.

Joe kept track—five more years, then four more, then three. When he retired in June 2019, Station 38 threw a party for him. He wore a white sash with the words I'M RETIRED on it in gold letters. His family celebrated with a cake shaped like an ambulance. Finally, Joe had made it.

When I joined the FDNY's Bureau of Emergency Medical Services in 2004, it was full of old hands like Joe. Not anymore. These days, people with Joe's experience are an endangered species. We have around 4,200 members, and maybe 5 percent have been on the job for fifteen years or more. The majority of emergency medical technicians and paramedics serving the public of New York City have less than five years' experience.

There's a reason for this. An EMT who makes $35,000 a year can't afford to live in the city. More than half of the younger medics at my EMS station live outside the five boroughs. I have a medic who comes in from Pennsylvania, another who lives in New Jersey. They wait tables or drive for Uber for extra cash. I'm a conditions boss, and even I work on the side—I moonlight as a paramedic at Aqueduct Racetrack on some days, and on other days I test defibrillators for a supplier. One of my colleagues has been in the service for twenty years and has a second job at a supermarket. Imagine: you work a crazy tour, dealing with heart attacks and broken limbs, and then you spend the evening stocking soup on aisle twelve.

I am forty-four years old. I've been in the service for nearly twenty years. I'm a dinosaur. But in my early days, people who had as much experience in EMS as I do now were a dime a dozen.

The guy who got me into the business had been in emergency medicine for nearly three decades when I met him in 2001. His name was Bill Simon. Bill had joined the force in the 1970s, right when the United States was developing its first national emergency medical system. He worked with the FDNY and took extra shifts on an ambulance at Maimonides Medical Center, a huge hospital in Borough Park, close to Station 40.

I got to know Bill when I was serving bagels in a store opposite the hospital. My life had gone off the rails—not that it had ever been fully on them. I grew up in 1980s Brooklyn, which in those days was dangerous, neglected, and a lot of fun. My parents were first- and second-generation Americans, with one foot in up-and-coming Park Slope and the other in the ghetto. They were practically kids themselves when they had Yvonne, my sister, and then my brother, Richie. I followed thirteen years behind him.

My family was middle class, if being middle class meant having salaried jobs and a car, owning property, and going on vacations to Disney World. At the same time, the Almojeras rolled around in the gutter with the best of Brooklyn's misfits and degenerates. Drugs, gambling, adultery, larceny—my family was into everything.

Despite this, I was an excellent student. Played basketball. I was fast-tracked in middle school and got a place at a selective high school in Manhattan. It looked like I might break with family tradition and actually graduate, maybe even go to college if my parents would cough up the cash.

But my family's dysfunction was biting at my heels. *Not so fast, young Anthony,* it said. *There's still time for things to fall apart.* And they did.

My father left when I was fourteen. He took off to live in Sheepshead Bay with a heroin addict who'd gone to high school with my sister. And then my brother, Richie—a troubled extrovert lost to criminality—was killed when I was sixteen years old.

The family crumbled. My mother stopped paying attention to me, to the properties she owned, to her finances. My father and his drug-addled girlfriend withdrew into their seedy life. My sister, Yvonne, retreated to Staten Island with her husband and their young family. She battened down the hatches.

I was still in high school; I wasn't in a position to take off somewhere and escape the Almojera chaos. I went from being a top student to skipping class and spending my days hanging at a friend's house. I would have flunked out except that my pride kicked in. I crammed in a ton of classes and graduated six months late.

After high school, I bounced around: Did a semester of college. Dropped out. Took acting classes. Got some gigs—*Titus Andronicus* at a playhouse in Queens, the hands in an ad for Palmolive soap.

By then, my temper had become explosive. When I was eighteen, Mom threw a bottle at my Datsun Maxima during an argument, so I rammed my car into hers (it was parked at the time). And it wasn't just family I fought with. I feel for anyone who crossed me in those days. When I was in my early twenties, a guy picked a fight with me over a parking spot, and I shoved his head into his windshield so hard that the glass cracked. I'd grown up around violence, and now that Richie was dead, it felt like the natural way to get my anger out.

One year after I finished high school, I landed a job in a bagel store in Park Slope. I stayed there for a few years. The bagel guys were crazy and alpha, and they looked after me. One was a former minor-league baseball player, one was a former boxer, one was a former drug dealer. And there was Marshall Johnson. Like me, Marshall was an aspiring actor. Unlike me, he was extremely good-looking and worldly and very successful with women. He was also a sex addict whose father had beaten him when he was a kid. We connected. We're still very close.

I dated a few girls. They didn't fall for me the way they did for Marshall or the way they had for Richie. But I enjoyed talking to women, and they seemed to appreciate my interest. I went out with a high-school friend for a couple of years. Her name was Marilyn. When I was twenty-two, she left me for another guy. That broke my heart.

It was after Marilyn dumped me that I first paid for sex. Some of the single guys at the bagel store did it. Even Marshall. He would browse the back pages of the *Village Voice*. The idea of paying a woman for sex felt wrong and it scared me. But I craved physical contact. I became curious.

Every day, I drove past the prostitutes on Third Avenue in Park Slope. One night, I pulled over. A woman in a pink halter top and a blond wig came over to the passenger-side window. She told me what she would do and what it would cost. She got into the car. I was so nervous that we didn't really do anything. In truth, it wasn't sex that I was after. It was affection. The feeling of being attractive.

After that fumble in my car, I started seeing women from an escort service. I saw the same women again and again. They would come to my apartment. We would talk. I'd make them cups of tea and ask them their real names. It helped me to feel like I wasn't just another john taking advantage of them. Even though, of course, I was.

After a few years at the bagel store, I got itchy feet. I was single, and my acting career was not taking off, so I decided to try my luck in Montana. I wanted to go somewhere wild and remote, and I'd been obsessed with Montana since childhood. In August 2000, I packed up my 1987 Ford Ranger pickup and headed west.

Montana was everything I had imagined: Open skies, horses. Snow. I rented a room in a house that didn't even have a lock on the front door. I got a job in—you guessed it—another bagel store. I made friends with a tracker named Zak Mercer who taught me how to tell a billy goat from a boulder a hundred yards away. I spent days hiking alone in Glacier National Park and the National Bison Range. The mountains there were snowcapped with big, jagged cliffs. They were created by so much violence, but they were two of the most beautiful places I had ever seen.

Still, I didn't fit in. I had grown up hopping the New York subway and break-dancing. In Brooklyn, a date involved going for a bite, then to a movie or maybe a play. In Montana, it involved activities like elk bugling, which Zak tried to teach me to do. Apparently, nothing attracts a Montana woman like covering yourself in elk urine and mimicking the call of a horny buck. I was a flop.

And I couldn't shake the anxiety that had eaten at me since Richie died. I was constantly on edge. I started listening to Rush Limbaugh on the radio just to have someone to be angry with.

So in May 2001, I returned to New York. The bagel store rehired me. Marshall and I moved into an apartment in Red Hook. We were living there when the World Trade Center collapsed. Red Hook is across the water from the tip of Manhattan, so we sat in the yard and looked at the plume of smoke on the other side of the bay. Sheets of Cantor Fitzgerald letterhead fell around us like leaves.

It wasn't long afterward that I joined EMS. I could lie and say that I was inspired by the sacrifices that members of the emergency services made on 9/11. But the truth was less poetic: The bagel guys sent me to work in their store in Borough Park, and when Bill Simon came in there, he told me stories about going into people's homes and zooming through New York streets, about the blood and the drama. I was fascinated. When there were no customers, I'd pull up a chair and ask Bill and his colleagues to tell me about their work. The more I heard, the more emergency services sounded like a job that would suit me. It didn't require a college degree. It came with a solid paycheck. And it would provide lots of raw emotion—a good thing for an actor, which was what I still aspired to be.

At first, I didn't think of EMS as a long-term job option. I planned to stay in it only until my acting career took off. But once I started helping people and running to emergencies, it became my life.

Emergency medical services had also become Joe's life. Which, right then, he was struggling to hold on to.

"Not the scoop," Joe said. "Anthony, I don't want to go on the scoop."

I knelt to speak to him. I had asked the medics on scene to get the scoop, which is a stretcher that splits lengthwise. If a patient has extremely low blood pressure, you cannot sit him up or let him stand, because the blood will drain from the vital organs in the upper body. You have to carry those patients on their backs.

"Joe, man. You know what we have to do," I said. "We can't get a reading on your blood pressure, it's so low. We have to lay you flat."

Things were not looking good. On my way up the stairs to Joe's apartment, I'd hoped that he was just having an episode of some sort. He drank a lot of coffee. He ate a lot of salty food. He had smoked for years before he quit. Maybe he'd had a minor stroke, I thought. But the minute I saw Joe on the floor, pouring sweat, I realized this was much more serious. The EKG indicated a posterior myocardial infarction. This happens when the tissue at the rear wall of the heart is deprived of oxygen, usually because a clot or a ruptured plaque is blocking an artery.

A posterior MI is a major emergency, but it's treatable. Many people survive. What worried me was that Joe's blood pressure was extremely low, and his heart rate was slowing.

Because Joe's heart wasn't getting enough oxygen, it wasn't pumping properly, and it wasn't maintaining pressure in his blood vessels, which meant that the rest of his body wasn't getting enough oxygen either. We could use a vasoconstrictor—in this case, dopamine—to increase pressure, but we needed authorization to give it to him. One of the medics called telemetry for permission.

While we waited for the go-ahead from telemetry, we split the scoop and slid the two sections under Joe, one on either side. We rolled him slightly to get him onto the two wings of the stretcher, then clipped the sides together.

Earlier, I had sent for an engine company and a second paramedic unit. Managing a patient who's having a heart attack requires a lot of hands, and I wanted resources—absolutely everything we could throw at the situation. One of the medic crews carried Joe down the stairs with his head tilted down so they could keep blood flowing to his heart, brain, and lungs. When we got him into the ambulance, his blood pressure was 60/40. An improvement, since earlier we hadn't been able to get a reading at all. But Joe was still circling the drain.

I put four paramedics in the back of the ambulance with Joe and followed with Serpil, his sister, in my truck. I turned down the volume on the radio so that she wouldn't hear what the paramedics were telling the hospital; I knew it would not be good.

I was worried. Very worried. When you're treating a gravely ill patient, you're always a bit scared. You need to be; it's what keeps you on your toes. But when you don't know the patient, there's some distance. This was different. I was rattled. I'd never expected to see Joe, with his coffee and his paunch, like this.

We headed to Maimonides, the hospital where Bill Simon had worked. Maimonides has one of the busiest emergency departments in the country. It's the Tower of Babel of health care. They say you can hear seventy languages there. It also happens to be one of the best hospitals in the country for heart-attack survival. The first heart transplant in the United States—the second in the world—was performed at Maimonides. This was the hospital for Joe.

I pulled up behind the ambulance in the emergency bay. When I opened the ambulance doors, the medics were pacing Joe's heart—sending measured electrical pulses through the wall of his chest to keep his heart beating. This was not a good sign. I reached for the stretcher to help pull him out. And that's when things got even more screwed up.

As I pulled out the stretcher, something I had done hundreds and hundreds of times, the damn thing malfunctioned. The stretcher tipped, with Joe on it. I lunged to catch it. A stretcher holding a two-hundred-pound man is too heavy to stop with one arm. I felt something snap. *What the hell was that?* I thought. I tumbled to the ground. Joe's sister told me later that I rolled over and over, like someone who'd jumped out of a train in a Western. I don't remember rolling. The pain was obliterating, I guess.

The medics rushed Joe into the emergency department. A cop helped me inside. An ED nurse gave me ice and put my arm in a sling.

Then Sara Lupin appeared. Sara's a close friend who was also a lieutenant paramedic. She'd joined Station 38 as a rookie paramedic when I was working there. We picked up overtime together and chased calls like crazy. Joe had been her lieutenant. Now Sara worked in the EMS Haz-Tac Battalion, which oversaw the teams that handled search and rescue and incidents involving hazardous materials. Rescue medics are nearly all male, but here was Sara, all five feet two inches of her, running the medical response at train derailments and building collapses. Yet when Sara heard that Joe had fallen sick, she'd asked to be assigned to help. Which was lucky for me; with one arm out of action, I needed a ride home.

"What happened?" Sara said. "Don't tell me you popped your biceps tendon! I had a boyfriend who did that. It's horrible."

Sara went to check on Joe while the nurse fixed up my arm. Then Sara pointed me in Joe's direction and went to fetch my truck. Joe was intubated, wires everywhere. Machines blinked and beeped all around him. Serpil and Dino were next to the bed. I stood beside Joe for a short while. Here we were, two hardened paramedics, one sick, one injured. Old dogs worn down by their profession.

I put my hand on Joe's. "It's going to be okay, Joe," I said. "You're going to be okay."

It felt strange to stand beside Joe patting his hand, trying to reassure him. Joe had been my mentor. I'd had several over the years, EMTs and paramedics who'd invested their time and energy in people they believed would stay in the profession. Joe had been a later influence, someone whose leadership style served as an example when I became a lieutenant paramedic. My first mentor, though, was Gregory Hodge.

Greg Hodge was my guide to Harlem. He walked me through my first assignment with the fire department. When I met Greg, I had been an EMT for a couple of years. I'd taken my first EMT qualification at a school in Flushing, Queens. It cost $650, and my dad had paid for the course.

Marshall had given up the apartment in Red Hook, and I couldn't afford the rent alone, so when I took the EMT course, I was homeless. I'd sold the Ford and bought a Nissan Pathfinder, which was where I slept. Every night, I drove to a dead-end street in Red Hook where I knew that the cops wouldn't bother me. I pushed the rear seats of the car down and spread a comforter across them. Then I climbed into my sleeping bag and opened my medical books.

I was a good EMS student. Scored over 90 in exams. Didn't have much interest in flash cards; I did better with the hands-on learning in the classroom. I qualified as an EMT in May 2002 and took a job doing medical transport in Staten Island. After work, I would drive my car a few blocks from the station and sleep in the back. Or, if I was the last person on the premises, I'd just curl up on the stretcher in the ambulance. I didn't want people to know I had nowhere to live.

Medical transport turned out to be unexciting and badly paid, nothing but elderly patients and dialysis patients. No emergencies. I enjoyed it, but what I really wanted was to work for the FDNY. The fire department runs emergency medical services for New York City. It's the biggest show in town. So I waited for a spot to open up at the FDNY Emergency Medical Services Academy.

Joining the FDNY meant I had to repeat EMT school. Even if you've qualified elsewhere, you have to do the academy's thirteen-week course. But at least the department paid me while I studied from February to April 2004. With my new salary, I rented a glorified studio apartment with intermittent heat in Borough Park.

I had a home for the first time in two years. I bought a philodendron with striped reddish leaves and an armchair with brown upholstery from IKEA. For the first few nights, I slept in the chair. Then Marshall bought me a futon. I've since moved to a bigger apartment, but I still have the chair and the plant.

Even though I was living in Brooklyn, I applied to work for the FDNY in Harlem. I'd grown up in the Brooklyn melting pot—Russian, Eastern European, Irish, Italian, Greek, Chinese, Black. To me, Harlem was the heart of Black urban America. Home to blues and jazz. Also home to poverty and drugs and gun violence and, thus, lots of emergencies. It sounded perfect.

I was assigned to FDNY EMS Station 13 on 136th Street and Lenox Avenue. It was part of the old Harlem Hospital building. Harlem in the early 2000s was on the cusp of becoming wealthier and whiter. There were people from other neighborhoods buying up the brownstones around St. Nicholas Park, a hilly strip that runs north from 128th Street. But the area was still mostly Black and mostly poor. The crack epidemic of the 1990s had wrecked the health of the community. People in Harlem were being murdered and dying of alcohol- and drug-related problems at very high rates. Even today, if you're born in central Harlem, you can expect to live a decade less than somebody born in Tribeca or SoHo, just a short subway ride to the south.

A few months after I arrived in Harlem, I joined Greg's unit. A unit consists of a group of EMTs or paramedics who divide the day into three eight-hour tours, or shifts, with three members assigned to each tour. Two of the three work on the ambulance while the third is off, so we each have two other people that we work with regularly, plus all the people we work alongside when we switch tours or pick up overtime.

Greg grew up in central Harlem, on the southern end of St. Nicholas Park. He had cheeks like a cherub and arched eyebrows that made him look permanently curious. He was a churchgoer, very intelligent, and in very good shape. He was also a former Delta Airlines pilot. He could have made a lot of money flying planes, but he wanted to serve his community, so he joined EMS.

I still remember our first day. Greg was in the driver's seat. "Anthony, I'll teach you all you need to know," he said. "But you must understand that when you're treating people between a Hundred and Tenth and a Hundred and Fifty-Fifth, you're treating my people."

Greg taught me medicine, for sure, but more important, he schooled me in how to be respectful and relaxed around people whose culture I didn't share. Showed me how to walk into a houseful of people who were scared or angry, people whose taboos were different than mine and whose understanding of medicine was different than mine, and put all of them at ease.

At first, I didn't get it. I thought that people would just let me do what I needed to do. I was the one with medical training, right? Wrong. You can't just march into strangers' homes and ask them to let you touch their bodies and stick things into them. Not everyone wants you there. Not everyone trusts you.

But Greg had a way with people. He was serene. He was polite but familiar. He had a lilting voice that made you feel relaxed. Greg would roll up a woman's sleeve to take her blood pressure as he asked, "Hey, Mrs. Robinson, how's your granddaughter?"

Even the way Greg walked was calm. I ran everywhere in those days—rushed to every call, sprang from the ambulance. Greg never even broke into a trot. But somehow, he always reached the patient as quickly as I did.

I didn't have much to offer Greg in the way of wisdom, but I did introduce him to one thing. We were dropping a patient at a midtown hospital one day and I suggested we go to the Carnegie Deli, which was just south of Central Park. Greg said he'd never been there. I couldn't believe it. I went all over the city as a kid. I went to Coney Island on the subway. I went to Yankee Stadium. When I was seven, I joined a break-dancing crew that took the F train each Saturday to dance in Times Square. I assumed that every kid in the city had grown up on a long leash like I had. But life wasn't like that for Greg. Kids from his part of town didn't venture south of 110th Street; that was where the white people lived. I realized then that looking like a white kid—even though I was half white, half Filipino—gave me freedom that other people didn't have.

We drove to the deli, and I bought Greg a pastrami sandwich that was stacked so high, it was hard to open your mouth wide enough to bite into it.

Greg munched and swallowed; he was very well mannered. Then he said, "Anthony, this is the best sandwich I have ever eaten."

For years, every time I saw Greg, he would say, "Remember when we went to the Carnegie Deli? Remember that sandwich?" And he would chuckle.

The beauty of those days was that EMTs like Greg took the time to show rookies like me the ropes. Another one of my partners was Henry Cabrera, a Dominican EMT from Washington Heights. He was in the same unit as Greg but worked a different tour; between trading shifts and working overtime, I spent a ton of time with them both. Henry sculpted his hair into a perfect shiny wave with gel. He had a sharp crease down each sleeve and each pants leg.

"You've always got to be squared away, brother," Henry would say. "There's going to be times when you don't know what is going on, and you're going to have to fake it. If you look professional, the family is not going to think twice."

Henry taught me to open front doors in Dominican neighborhoods gently, without pushing them all the way. Many families keep a bowl of camphor water behind the door to ward off bad spirits. A few months after he told me that, I was working with a rookie EMT in Harlem, and he barged into a Dominican home and knocked over the water. The old lady shook her head and refused to let us treat her.

When it came to finding the angles, my best teacher was Norman Gillard, Stormin' Norman. He was another EMT from Harlem. Big guy, former military. Norman was good-looking and had the distinction—and still does, to this day—of being allowed to wear a short beard. Facial hair is a no-no in EMS, but Norman convinced the fire department to let him keep his. He would rub oil between his palms and run his fingers through the curls.

Norman was wily. He taught me how to work the system by swapping shifts with other EMTs so that everyone ended up with a convenient schedule, what we call "doing a mutual." Mutuals are key to freeing up time for family or the many gigs that medics work on the side to make extra money. Norman also taught me to give my colleagues a heads-up if I was going to bang out—in other words, call in sick. "Listen here, cat," he said. "When you're gonna bang out, make sure you tell your people first. Then they can pick up the over-time."

Like Greg, Norm had a way with patients. His specialty was female patients. He was also good with family members. I recall walking into an apartment building with Norman to pick up an elderly woman. Her son was very agitated, asked what had taken us so long. He was aggressive. He made me nervous. But there was a fantastic smell coming from the kitchen. Something frying.

Norm stuck his head in the kitchen and asked for a plate of food. Just like that. Then, without waiting, he got Grandma out of bed, helped her dress, put her in the wheelchair. We were about to leave the apartment when a woman appeared with a plate of plantains for Norman. As we rolled Grandma into the elevator, she was clutching Norm's food.

When it came to medicine, my EMT partners in Harlem knew that the only way to learn was to get your hands dirty. You can deliver a thousand plastic babies, but you won't be effective until you've held a slimy newborn head in your hands, felt the umbilical cord throbbing and the tiny pulse that's still flowing from the mother to the baby, then cut the baby free for its first independent breath. Learn all you want from textbooks and classroom demonstrations, but until you feel it and smell it and see it, you don't know a thing.

I'd been up in Harlem for about a month when I went on a call for a woman in labor with an EMT named Calvin Smith. Smitty wasn't my usual partner, but I was working overtime. It was a weekend night, around eleven. Smitty and I pulled up at a housing project around 125th and Amsterdam in Harlem. We got into the elevator and were heading up to the ninth floor when I began to feel nervous. In EMT school, we'd gotten lectures on childbirth. We'd practiced with dummies. But I'd never seen a real birth.

"Smitty," I said. "You ever deliver a baby?"

Smitty gave me a look that said, *Is the pope Catholic?* He wasn't a man of many words.

I relaxed a little. *Smitty's got this,* I thought. I figured we'd probably take the patient to the hospital, and if it was too late for the hospital, I'd get to stand back and watch my first delivery.

Wrong and wrong.

We rang the doorbell. A man in his late thirties answered. He ushered us down a hallway. As we passed the living room, I noticed a bunch of kids sitting around, some on the couch, some on the floor. They were his children, the man said. Seven in all.

The woman was lying in the bedroom, propped up on a pile of pillows. Her knees were bent. A sheet was stretched across them like a tent. It was a spacious room. On one side of the bed there was a wooden dresser with a large television on top of it. There was a pile of clothes on the floor. The father sat down in a small, worn armchair.

"Hi," I said. "I'm Anthony."

I put the equipment bag down next to the bed and reached for the emergency obstetrical kit. Smitty walked to the corner of the room and stationed himself there. *Wait!* I thought. *You're going to leave this to me?* I shot a look in his direction. I knew better than to say anything. In emergency medicine—in any kind of patient care—you don't discuss your doubts in front of patients. Smitty raised his eyebrows and chuckled quietly. *You got this,* he was saying.

I took a breath. I started asking the woman questions. How many weeks pregnant was she? When was her last menstrual cycle? When was she due? If we have a patient who is in labor, we need to know how far along the pregnancy is. A thirty-two-week baby presents a very different situation than a forty-week baby. Premature babies may not be able to breathe on their own or maintain their body temperature. They need immediate neonatal intensive care.

"I'm due around now," the woman said.

"How far apart are your contractions?" I asked.

"Five or six minutes."

"Great!" I said. A surge of relief.

"Great?" The woman looked incredulous. "What do you mean, great?"

"Er . . . well, we have lots of time," I said. My understanding was that five or six minutes between contractions meant the birth was an hour away, maybe more. We could get the mother into the ambulance and take her over to St. Luke's Roosevelt on 114th Street.

"Honey," she said, "this baby is coming. We ain't got no time."

Then she made a little *o* with her lips and started to puff. Another contraction.

I glanced again at Smitty. This was the moment for him to step in. But Smitty didn't budge. I was on my own.

My heart was in my throat. I did a mental rehearsal of what we'd learned at the academy. *If the baby is presenting head-down, apply a little pressure to the crown to prevent it bursting out too quickly and causing tears; use a downward movement to deliver the anterior shoulder and an upward one for the posterior. The rest of the body should follow.*

I knew I had to make sure the umbilical cord wasn't wrapped around the baby's neck, knew to suction mucus from the nose and mouth. I knew to clamp and then cut the cord at a point at least four finger-widths from the woman's vagina and the baby's belly. And I knew to wait for the delivery of the full placenta, which I would put in a special red bag.

The husband sat in his chair, resting his chin on his fist. He looked almost bored. I realized I was the novice in the room. Smitty had delivered plenty of babies. The woman had given birth to seven children. The father had seen it all. I was the only one who had no clue what I was doing.

The woman kept puffing, short, fast breaths. I lifted the sheet slightly and helped her remove her underwear. She was sweating. I was sweating. I pushed the sheet up to her hips. She let her thighs fall wide apart. Peeping from her vagina was a small triangle of hair. I thought I was going to pass out.

The woman groaned and dug her heels into the bed. I took a long breath. *Come on, Anthony,* I thought. *You have to guide the head.*

I placed my hand below the protruding crown. The mother screamed, and the head slithered out, then the shoulders, just like that. A baby boy shot straight into my gloved hands.

By this point, the father had stirred himself and was up by the mother's head, stroking her cheek and smiling. Smitty stood silently in the corner. I clamped the umbilical cord and cut it.

And then I just stood there, staring at the baby and thinking, *The first person to hold you in this world is me.*

. . .

In Harlem, I became a buff. It's the word we use for a medic who gets down, who chases jobs, who says that he's close to the emergency and can be there in the blink of an eye even when he's forty blocks away. Some medics sit in the outfield and hope that the ball won't come their way. Not me. I play the infield. I want the ball.

I'd always wanted to be a superhero. I grew up collecting comic books—Green Lantern, the Flash. In the living room of my apartment in central Brooklyn, I have statuettes of Wonder Woman and Superman. I have a green plastic lamp, a working green lantern, in my bedroom. And even now, when I hit the siren and feel people staring—maybe shuddering at the thought they could be next—I feel the cape billowing from my shoulders.

About nine months after I started at Station 13, two awesome new EMTs joined my unit: Phil Jungenheimer and Mike Suehle. Phil was a former Marine; Mike had been a combat medic. Both loved to get down. The ambulance that Phil, Mike, and I worked became one of the busiest in the division. Our call sign was Eleven Frank. We would jump on every emergency: "Eleven Frank, two minutes out." It didn't matter where we were; we always said we were two minutes away. We'd squeal to a stop at the scene of the emergency, brake pads smoking, and jump down from the ambulance into an acrid cloud.

And like every good EMT, I was baptized in blood. One day, several months into the job, I was with Phil in the ambulance bay at New York–Presbyterian on 168th and Broadway. A report of a shooting came over the radio: Three people down. Corner of 125th and Frederick Douglass Boulevard—well outside our range.

I looked at Phil. His eyes lit up.

"Let's go," I said.

We sped down Broadway and reached the scene in about four minutes. We grabbed one of the wounded men and put him in the bus. He'd been shot in the right side of the chest and had a hemopneumothorax—air and blood were entering the chest cavity from the gunshot wound, and the lung had collapsed. He also had a wound in his neck. Blood spurted from his carotid artery and spattered on my face and chest.

We got him to the hospital, and I watched as the trauma team tried to save our patient. A doctor made an incision on one side of the man's rib cage. Into it, she inserted a chest tube—a plastic tube about the width of two fingers—and used it to remove air and blood from the chest cavity so the lung could reinflate. The team used a thumper, a machine that performed CPR, to do chest compressions.

But they couldn't get a pulse.

About ten minutes after we arrived in the ED, the doctors pronounced the man dead. They peeled away to other emergencies. The nurses began to remove the wires and instruments that were attached to the patient.

Even though we had lost the guy, the effort to save him amazed me. I was hooked. As I left the trauma bay, I bumped into Stormin' Norman. My face was caked with blood. Blood had soaked into my uniform and was all over my arms.

"Look at you, cat," said Norm. He nodded with appreciation. "You ain't a rookie no more."

During the Harlem years, I began to build my surrogate family, the circle of friends I call the Group Home because we're all misfits or people who've been abandoned in one way or another.

One of the founding members was Mike Sullivan, who I met in 2004 when Mike was an EMT at a different Harlem station than mine. (Mike later became a senior paramedic and worked in the Bronx.) At the time, he, too, was an aspiring actor. Mike saw me reading the *New York Times* in the emergency department while I waited to transfer a patient. He complimented me on it. He was a bit of an intellectual— studied at the Boston Conservatory. We hit it off.

Mike and I started working overtime together and hanging out outside of work. We would watch baseball together, even though Mike was a Boston fan. We'd go out to eat, go to plays. I'd talk about women I liked, and he'd talk about men. Mike had been dating a good-looking but complicated guy when I met him, but the pair broke up soon after we became friends. We shared some ground—when Mike was eight, he, too, had lost a brother. A freak accident. His brother, who was ten years older than him, was electrocuted while he was working in a dairy.

The Group Home would prove to be my family of choice, the circle of friends who looked out for me and for one another. We traveled together, spent the holidays together, went to one another's family funerals. The group absorbed my long-standing friends, like my bagel-shop buddy Marshall, and grew over the years to include many Brooklyn-based medics. But it started in Harlem with Mike.

I loved everything about Harlem and being an EMT there. But it didn't take long for me to understand that paramedics had more fun. The medics up in Harlem let EMTs try procedures that we weren't trained or authorized to do. They'd be putting an IV in a patient and they'd let me try to find the vein and get the needle in. They showed me how to use a laryngoscope, taught me how to find the little white V of the vocal cords in the throat. I was amazed—still am—by how patient patients were. They let me prod and poke in the wrong places because they knew I needed to learn.

Barely a year after I joined the FDNY, I signed up for the paramedic training program. It was grueling. Nine months of night school, emergency department rotations, psych rotations, ride-alongs, and exams. I sold my Pathfinder to pay for the course. After graduating in August 2005, I was assigned to Station 38 in East Flatbush, Brooklyn. And that was where I met Joe.

About a month before Joe's heart gave out, I bumped into him at Villabate Alba, an old-school Italian pastry store on Eighteenth Avenue in

Bensonhurst. When I was a kid, my parents would go there to buy my birthday cakes. The bakery also had the best gelato in Brooklyn. It was a gorgeous late-September evening. I had just returned from a trip to Uganda with Mike and Angie Alburquerque, another member of the Group Home.

Joe was on one of his walks. He walked all over Brooklyn. He would walk from Bay Ridge to Brighton Beach and back, a six-mile loop. He loved the city, and now that he was retired, he had time to enjoy it.

Joe ordered espresso. He asked about my trip to Africa. We'd gone to the Maasai Mara and Uganda and Zanzibar, I told him. We'd seen rhinos and volunteered on a project, digging wells.

"Jeez, Anthony," he said. "You haven't changed. You don't rest on these vacations!" Joe always teased me because he thought my trips were too ambitious.

He drained his espresso. We agreed to go for drinks before he went to North Carolina. I offered him a ride home.

"Thanks," Joe said. "But it's nice out. I think I'll walk."

NOVEMBER 2019

The Fire Department of New York's Emergency Medical Services Station 40 sits on one of the main drags of Sunset Park in central Brooklyn. A neighborhood of brick and limestone houses and low-rise apartment buildings, Sunset Park is edged by disused piers that stick out into the water like the teeth of a broken comb. At its center is a well-kept park with an outdoor swimming pool. The park is one of the highest points in Brooklyn, and there are long benches there where I like to watch the sun go down over the harbor. You can see Manhattan across the water. It looks like the Emerald City.

Sunset Park has large Asian and Latino communities. To the west of the station are bodegas and taco joints and Mexican bakeries. You hear *cumbia* floating from the cars. The neighborhood slopes toward the waterfront under the Brooklyn-Queens Expressway and turns cobbled and industrial.

To the east of the station are Chinese banks, herbalists, seafood markets, acupuncturists, jewelers. Every EMS station gets to design its own logo, and ours has two dragons facing each other breathing fire. Outside, we have a yellow neon sign with the number 40, designed to look like Chinese calligraphy.

On one side of Station 40 is a senior citizens' center—a large room with a linoleum floor and rows of white plastic tables. A few years ago, I started popping in to play mah-jongg. The players are mainly women. "We play for money," they warned me. My opponent bet me a quarter. She won. She won again. The women always beat me, but I keep playing.

On the other side of the station is a Chinese bakery that sells chicken feet and dim sum and coconut buns filled with cream. I don't know any Mandarin and the staff doesn't know much English, so I point at the dim sum and that's how we get by. I once went to the bakery with a former ambulance partner, Doraun Ellis, who had learned Mandarin and Spanish. Doraun was very studious. He covered his books with duct tape because he didn't want his coworkers to judge him by what he read. Doraun ordered in Mandarin, and everyone stared. A tall Black guy speaking their language—they were so happy.

Station 40 used to be a firehouse, and it has giant red doors with a regular-size door cut out of them; it looks like the entrance to a castle. The doors open onto the apparatus floor, which is basically a cave where a fire truck once stood. Hanging from the ceiling, there's a flag of honor bearing the names of the 343 FDNY members who died in the 9/11 attacks, a New York State flag, and a blue-and-white banner celebrating my fellow EMS lieutenant Joe McWilliams. In 2017, Joe ran into a burning building down the street and pulled people out. The fire department awarded Joe a leadership medal. We were proud. It's not often that the fire department recognizes the work that the medical side does. (Heroism seems to run in his family; Joe's brother Dan was one of the firefighters who famously lifted the flag at Ground Zero after the World Trade Center attacks.)

The walls of Station 40 are lined with red cages for service members to stow their belongings, their bulletproof vests, and their tech bags— red duffels full of the medical equipment that every EMT or paramedic must carry. There's a supply room where we keep advanced-life-support equipment and nonnarcotic drugs. (Narcotics are kept in a safe with two locks; nobody ever carries both sets of keys.) There are drums of diesel exhaust fluid; shovels and salt for the snow; a couple of bicycles; and some tall potted plants that overwinter indoors. It's charming in its way, but it's an awkward space for a medical team that doesn't have a fire truck. We're squeezed into offices upstairs and a room in the back that has whiteboards and a television and two old couches.

I think of the layout of Station 40, with its huge space for a non-existent fire truck, as a metaphor for the status of EMS in the fire department. We're kind of an afterthought, the product of a 1996 merger between the fire department and the emergency medical services division of the New York City Health and Hospitals Corporation. Except *merger* suggests a marriage of equals, whereas this was more of a colonization of EMS by the fire department. FDNY has more than ten thousand uniformed service members; EMS has about forty-two hundred. Plus, the fire department has a more established culture. Every firefighter seems to have a father or an uncle who was a firefighter. EMS is a younger profession, with people from a mixture of backgrounds. Nobody I know claims to come from three generations of paramedics.

Besides, firefighters have a sacred place in the public imagination. When people see a shiny fire truck, their eyes get wide. When they see an ambulance, they look away. To acknowledge us is to acknowledge the frailty of life, the fact that you're just a sack of bones, and someday one of those bones is going to break.

For the fire department, merging with EMS was a way to stay relevant and generate income. There are fewer fires these days than there were thirty years ago. Fire codes are stricter, and prevention is better. But the general population has become older, so there are more medical emergencies. Rather than downsize, the fire department took on more medical work—a shift that happened in many American cities, not just New York.

On the top floor of the station, we have a gym with benches and old weight machines. Nothing fancy. There's a flat roof that looks out over Brooklyn South, our area of responsibility. Brooklyn South falls into FDNY EMS Division 5, which covers part of Brooklyn and Staten

Island. (The city is carved into nine divisions, all of which have several EMS stations, each led by an EMS captain.) I often think about making a garden on the roof. I love the view—streets and streets that stretch to the ocean across a landscape that's as flat as a plate. Borough Park, Bensonhurst, Mapleton, Gravesend, Dyker Heights, Fort Hamilton, Bay Ridge. Tire-repair shops. Lebanese falafel joints. Adventist churches. There aren't many tourists other than the people who go to Coney Island to sit on the beach or ride the Cyclone. It's not the Brooklyn you see in movies and real estate ads. But for me and my patients, it's home.

When I am on duty at the station—we call it "sitting the desk"—I work in a corner of the apparatus floor in a brick cubicle with windows. The cubicle resembles a subway ticket booth. There are computers and a monitor where the status of each ambulance is shown by color: red for units that are on scene; yellow for units on their way to a call; green for those en route to the hospital. There's the 400 MHz radio for communicating with Dispatch and another radio on an 800 MHz frequency that EMS officers use to communicate among themselves. There are calendars and clipboards with the rundown of each ambulance tour. There's a record of crew members' exposure to potentially dangerous biological substances. Files where we log tests on our glucometers and supplies of narcotics and equipment that's out for repair. There are canisters of WD-40, which we use mostly to get broken keys out of ambulance locks and ignitions. There's a space heater and a television.

If it's very quiet on a Sunday or a night tour, I stream David Attenborough documentaries. I find them calming. Humans can be so perverse; we screw each other up. The way that wild animals live makes more sense to me.

My attraction to nature inspired me to become a Buddhist in my thirties. The natural world is where a Buddhist feels most at peace, ready for enlightenment. If I could, I'd meditate under a tree every day. But that's not easy in the center of Brooklyn, so I make do with the altar in the corner of my bedroom.

Most of the time, though, the station is pretty lively. Ambulance crews come in to pick up supplies or change their uniforms or heat up their lunches. When they're not on calls, they park at designated intersections referred to as eighty-nines. The intersections are dotted around South Brooklyn so our units are evenly spread out. The area outside our station is cramped, so even if it made tactical sense for everyone to park here, there'd be no way to do it.

But on Thanksgiving, everyone's allowed to hang at the station, at least for a few hours. Nobody gets kicked out on my watch. And Thanksgiving is always my watch. I'm single more often than not, and I have no kids, so I offer to work. It saves me from worrying about who I'm going to spend the holidays with.

At the station, we organize a potluck dinner, watch the football game. Ambulance crews come and go. Thanksgiving is a popular day for heart attacks and the like, because members of the public eat and drink too much. In fact, the evening before Thanksgiving is usually one of the busiest nights of the year. It seems folks like to get trashed before they spend the day with their families.

When I was a kid, my family always made a big deal of the holidays. We painted eggs for Easter. On St. Patrick's Day, my mom baked Irish soda bread. For Thanksgiving, she gathered the family: her mom; Richie; Richie's girlfriend, Holly; and their son, Anthony (I was named after my paternal grandfather; little Anthony was named after Holly's dad). My sister, Yvonne, would be there and, in later years, my other nephew, Eddie.

I was closer in age to my nephews than my siblings. Yvonne was sixteen when I was born; Richie was thirteen. Richie and Holly's son, Anthony, came along when I was four, and Eddie was born when I was eight. By fourth grade, I was an uncle twice over.

From Dad's side of the family, Mom invited Aunt Marion and Uncle Dominic. Marion and Dominic were separated. Marion was my dad's sister. She was small and brash, but fun. She worked at the amusement park at Coney Island, and she would slip me a wristband so I could ride the Cyclone for free. Dominic had been handsome when he was young, a merchant marine with wavy hair and a gold tooth. Now all his teeth were shot from the heroin and methadone he used. I found him pretty skeevy. Mom and Dad said that Marion had ruined Dominic, that Marion was a whore. (A "huw-er" was how Mom said it.) I don't know how much truth there was to that, but there was no doubt that Marion had plenty of kids—seven in all—and only a couple were Dominic's.

Usually, some of Marion's kids came to Thanksgiving too—Mimi, Donna, Tuffy. They were closer in age to my siblings than me. Tuffy had fallen out of a third-floor window when he was three and hadn't cried. That's how he got his name. Mimi was my favorite. She was dark-haired and sweet and funny.

Even though Mom wasn't much of a cook, she and Yvonne would prepare a big spread: Turkey with all the trimmings. Extra turkey necks for my dad and me. Penne salad. Everyone would settle in the living room and watch the Cowboys and eat spinach dip, just like other families.

At Christmas, Mom would cover the house with colored lights. She had old lights with big, screw-in bulbs and muted colors. She would arrange them on the front of the house in the shape of a Christmas tree. I would climb onto the roof and dangle them over the eaves, and Mom would lean out of the upstairs window and fix them in place. She'd put tinsel in the bushes outside. Our house was the most decorated on the block.

We spent Christmas morning at home opening our gifts. Lots of gifts. Later, we drove to Lynbrook on Long Island to see my mom's sister Mary Jo; her husband, Walter; and their two kids. They lived in a big house with a fireplace and a yard. They had a golden retriever.

Walter was cheating on Mary Jo, but I didn't know that back then. To me, the family seemed perfect, like the families I saw on television.

The best thing about the holidays was that the fighting stopped. Some families save their arguments for Thanksgiving. The Almojeras did the opposite. We fought all year and then called a truce for a couple of days. We came out of the trenches and kicked a soccer ball and exchanged cigarettes. It was partly for the benefit of the guests, but mostly it was genuine. My parents just wanted us all to be nice to one another.

I imagine the fighting started the day my parents met in 1957. Linda Krings and Richard Almojera. They were high-schoolers in Hell's Kitchen. Mom was thirteen, Dad sixteen.

They were both new to the city. Mom had moved from Baltimore with her siblings, her mother—a hard woman and a hard drinker whose parents had immigrated from County Cork in Ireland—and her step-father, Frank, a short-order cook who molested my mother for years.

Dad's family had come to New York City from New Orleans. His father, Victor, was a ship's cook from the Philippines. He was in and out of port, in and out of family life. Much as my dad would be. By all accounts, Victor was very easygoing—unlike Eula, Dad's mom, who was manipulative and mean-spirited. When my father spent time in jail for robbery as a teenager, she tore up the letters my mother wrote him and told him that Mom had met another man.

I found Eula terrifying. We sometimes visited her in her apartment in Park Slope after Victor died. She had a deep raspy voice and a mustache, and she would sit on the edge of her canopy bed with her nylons wrinkled around her knees. She spoke to me in Creole. *"Prends!"* she'd say. Then she'd thrust a lollipop at me and kiss my cheek with her wet lips.

Dad had had a girlfriend when he met my mother. Not that Mom let that discourage her. She challenged the girl to a fight and won, or so the story goes. Mom didn't know that she'd be fighting women for my dad for the rest of his life.

Linda and Richard dated for a couple of years and then married. They had Yvonne in 1961 and Richie three years later. They rented an apartment in Park Slope. My father worked on the docks in Red Hook and Sunset Park, first loading and unloading containers and later as an electrician on the ships. He was gone for months at a time. My mother became a nurse's aide in the Madonna Residence, a nursing home near Prospect Park. In 1976, they bought a narrow house with a bay window on Thirteenth Street. The next year, I was born.

The map of my childhood was compact. I was born a few blocks from home at New York Methodist Hospital in Park Slope, baptized at Holy Family Church, opposite our house, and went to elementary school at PS 124, a grand limestone building on the corner of my street.

Until I was six, we lived in the house with the bay window. Mom and Dad slept in the same room. If I had a bad dream, they would tuck me in bed between them. When I was six, we moved to a bigger house a few doors away and my parents started sleeping apart—one in the bedroom and one on the recliner downstairs.

Around the time that we moved, Richie bought me a transistor radio. My family listened to music all the time. Jazz, gospel, blues. On Friday nights, I listened to hip-hop on DJ Red Alert's show. It started around eleven. I would tape the show on my cassette recorder. At the time, Richie was living at our house with Holly and little Anthony. If I fell asleep before the show started, he'd creep in and press the Record button for me. Richie could be sweet when he wasn't getting high.

After we moved to the house up the street, my parents gave our first house to Yvonne. She lived there with her husband, Eddie, and then with little Eddie, their son.

When I visited Yvonne, she fixed me food and we played Rummy 500. Eddie was a good guy—a corrections officer—but he was a lump on a log, so Yvonne went dancing on Fridays without him. I would watch as she and her friends put on makeup and sprayed their hair with Aqua Net. Yvonne was pretty, with arched eyebrows and long brown hair. She left Eddie for a guy named Joe—who's now her husband—when

I was nine. She rented a van and made off with all the furniture that she and Eddie owned. She also cleared out my mother's bank account. After that, I didn't see Yvonne as often, even when Richie was alive.

My best friends growing up, Christopher Chen and Anthony Rivera, lived on our block. We played a game called coco-levio that involved capturing members of an opposing team and putting them in jail (on the stoop, maybe). We climbed onto the roof of Holy Family and hid behind the parapet. We hung out on Chris's stoop.

Chris was on the heavy side and quite shy. His parents were hoarders. They had lumber stacked two feet high in the hallways and a tub in the bathroom stuffed with a hundred toothbrushes. They liked me. They knew that I studied and steered clear of drugs. They cooked Chinese food, and Chris and I would sit on a low bench in the living room and eat, surrounded by all their junk.

Chris and Anthony and I remained friends long after we left school. Chris got a job in information technology. When I was at the FDNY academy getting my EMT certificate, he gave me around three thousand dollars, maybe more, to tide me over. He was a very generous friend. A few years later, he called me and said he didn't feel good. I was a paramedic by then. I went to his house and took his blood pressure. It was 210/180, which is a hypertensive emergency. Blood pressure that high can damage organs and blood vessels.

"Chris, man, you need to go to the hospital," I said. "This is very serious."

But he wouldn't go. He had no insurance. A couple of months later, he keeled over at his desk in Manhattan, and that was that. I don't think I've ever missed anyone the way I miss Chris.

Now, only the Anthonys were left. But Anthony Rivera developed epilepsy, and he refused to take his meds. For a couple of years in the mid-2000s, he lived with me. I enjoyed his company, but I caught him stealing from me and I had to kick him out. Then, in 2017, Anthony had a prolonged seizure. I heard from a mutual friend that at the time, he was alone in the Brooklyn apartment that he shared with another guy. We'd lost touch by then, though, and I never found out anything more—only that he didn't make it.

I treat patients like Chris and Anthony all the time, people who will mostly likely die of preventable diseases because they don't have insurance or they can't afford their meds or simply don't take them. Neglect and poor mental health don't make for long lives.

Survival rates in my family weren't so high either. My older cousins—the ones who used to come to Thanksgiving—all died young. Aunt Marion's daughter Donna died of AIDS when I was twelve; Mimi, her other daughter, died of HIV-associated pneumonia. Marion's son Tuffy got into a fight with a local guy when he was in his twenties—I still don't know why—and the guy stabbed him to death. Marion herself lost a leg to diabetes and died in the early 2000s, not long after Mimi.

Even my nephew little Eddie—Yvonne's son, a gentle soul—made it to only twenty-nine. He got into bodybuilding and took steroids. I warned him off them, but he didn't listen. The steroids destroyed his immune system, and in 2014, Eddie developed pneumonia. They found him dead in his bed.

The New York that Chris and Anthony and I grew up in was a little crazy, but people looked out for one another. You knew the grocer by name; you knew the mailman. If you got out of line, a neighbor would give you a smack. Our next-door neighbor Mr. Chen (no relation to Chris) paid me to shovel his snow. Another neighbor, Mr. Haas, grew grapes over a pergola in his backyard. He was Greek. In the late summer, he would ask me to help him collect the grapes, then he would stuff the grape leaves and bring them to us on a plate.

Mom knew everybody in the neighborhood—the old folks, the punks, the women, the addicts. Even the guy who killed Tuffy. When the man was released from jail, he moved into an apartment that was a block from our house. Mom would stop and say hello. Looking back,

I assume that she knew something about how that fight went down. That Tuffy started it, perhaps. Even so, not every aunt would have found it in her heart to say hello to her nephew's killer.

Mom organized the block party with the church across the street; she got teams together to play softball. She ran a hustle at her bingo games, Fridays at St. Thomas Aquinas and Saturdays at the Fifth Avenue bingo hall. The players who were in on Mom's hustle would play the official bingo game with everyone else and make side bets on a different set of numbers. Mom would take a cut.

On summer evenings, Mom would sit in a metal lawn chair on the wide section of sidewalk opposite our house with my godmother, Kathy, and their friend Ruthie Salmon. They would conceal their Budweisers in paper bags. They'd talk about people in the neighborhood and drink their beer through straws.

I used to find it strange that people saw the shit that happened in my household—the hole in the wall where my dad ripped out the phone during a fight; my bandaged fourteen-year-old hand after I punched a plate-glass door—and yet still came to visit. There were barbecues in the backyard. Kathy came every day for a cup of tea. Whatever was going down in my house was going down in theirs too.

And Mom's social energy was infectious. I know I caught it. Over the years, my core of close friends, the so-called Group Home, has grown to include more than a dozen people. Most of them are medics. I'm the common denominator, the organizer. Barbecues, whitewater rafting, a trip to Dublin. I'm usually the one who comes up with the plan and gets people to come along.

A few weeks after Joe collapsed, I took an eight-day trip to Beijing and Hong Kong with some of my Group Home friends. Terence Lau, a medic who started out on my ambulance at Station 38, was born in Hong Kong. He'd left in the late 1980s to come to New York, and he hadn't been back. When we were partners, I promised to go with him to Hong Kong whenever he wanted. And earlier that year, he'd decided he was ready.

It felt like a strange time to go on vacation. My arm was no longer in a sling, but I had a brace on my elbow. Sara Lupin had guessed right: my distal biceps tendon—the tendon that attaches the muscle in your upper arm to your elbow—had snapped. Because part of the biceps was unattached, the muscle was useless. I had to use other muscles—in my shoulders, neck, forearm—to bear weight. I couldn't lift anything heavy.

And I was still very raw from what had happened to Joe.

Three days after Joe fell sick, I returned to the hospital. He had multi-organ failure and was on ECMO—extracorporeal membrane oxygenation. An ECMO machine oxygenates your blood and pumps it back into your body when your own heart and lungs can't do it. There was very little blood circulating to Joe's legs, and the doctors told me that he would lose one of them.

He was spared that indignity, at least. Joe died the next day.

Joe wouldn't have approved of me flying off to Hong Kong. *Another of your busy vacations!* he'd have said. But I needed distraction. And I'd found a bargain—three days in Beijing and five in Hong Kong for about nine hundred dollars, including flights.

Angie was in. Angie's also a medic. She has a wide, beautiful smile and a husky laugh. Her arms are covered in tattoos and her legs have scars from fighting as a kid. She's thirteen years younger than me, and I consider Angie my sister. (Like me and Mike, Angie lost an older brother when she was a kid; he was killed in a motorcycle accident.)

Kala, Angie's roommate, was also down for the trip. Angie and I had met Kala at Coachella a couple of years earlier. She was in her late twenties, from California. After she met us, she moved to New York to start law school with the goal of working in human rights law.

Raj, an old friend who was married to one of our medic buddies, came too. And so did Manny, a guy who worked in mental health at Lincoln Medical Center in the Bronx. Manny had joined the Group Home a few years earlier; he was very funny, very chill. Andres Segovia—Dre, we called him—came along as well. He was a medic in the Bronx who I'd met at the EMS academy. Ecuadoran. Very handsome.

In short, we were quite a crowd.

In Beijing, we saw the sights: the Great Wall, the Forbidden City, the Olympic Park. I'd been to China twice before, so I had seen them all, but it was fun to go back with people who hadn't.

On the third day, we flew to Hong Kong. There were huge protests outside our hotel, thousands of people chanting. People had been demonstrating for months against Beijing's grip on the former British territory. They were afraid of losing their freedoms. It was hard to breathe outside, there was so much tear gas and smoke. So we watched the demonstrations from our hotel window.

The next day we met up with Terence, who had flown to Hong Kong ahead of us. The protests were still going on, but we were able to get around. I'd been to Hong Kong before, so I got to play tour guide—Victoria Peak; the Tian Tan Buddha.

Terence took us to the massive white-and-spearmint-green apartment building where he had grown up. It's in the Ping Shek Estate, a huge public-housing project. Very impressive. Then we went to meet his grandma at a hole-in-the-wall restaurant in Kowloon. She was four feet tall and ninety years old. She had all her teeth. We joked with Terence about how Chinese people age slowly—his grandma was proof, we said. She was a live wire.

It felt great to be in a foreign city with friends. And even better, with local people who welcomed us and showed us all the best places to eat. At dinner with Terence's grandma, we ate tripe and chicken gizzards. Manny and Angie and Dre were wide-eyed when they saw the food, which was nothing like Chinese takeout in the Bronx.

I tried the cold winter-melon soup, just to be polite. Rule number one of travel is that you eat what your host offers you. It was revolting. I screwed up my face, and all of Terence's relatives laughed.

· · ·

It wasn't just Mom's sociability that rubbed off on me. I think I got some of her industriousness too. I got my first job in fifth grade. A truck would drop the *Daily News* at my house at about five a.m. and I'd load the copies into a shopping cart and deliver them all by seven thirty. I made about eighty dollars a week, a fortune for a ten-year-old. I would take my earnings, ride the D train by myself to Yankee Stadium, buy a bleacher ticket and a soda, and settle in for the game.

I was a pretty devoted sports fan—baseball, basketball, football. Even soccer. I watched ABC's *Wide World of Sports* every weekend and became hooked on Manchester United. When I was eight, Mom enrolled me in the fan club. I'm a member to this day.

Sometimes Mom would come with me to watch the Yankees. Not Dad; he didn't see the logic of paying for a game you could watch for free on television. So Mom and I would watch the game together and talk about the players—who had the best batting average, who was cute. We didn't fight. We didn't talk about Dad or Yvonne or even Richie. For a full nine innings, I had her all to myself.

Dad and I spent time together at home. He was friendly, but he wasn't social like my mom. When he wasn't working or at the offtrack betting place around the corner, Dad was in his home office next to the master bedroom, learning to program computers from a fat manual, taking a radio apart and putting it back together, playing chess against himself. Richie was the same; he took apart car engines and fixed ham radios. Richie paid attention to what Dad was doing. I didn't, but I liked to sit with him. We made model ships together and sometimes he'd help me with my homework.

When I was around eight years old, Dad and I would go to Manhattan on Sundays. We would walk up and down Canal Street and look in the electronics stores, then we'd go to Wo Hop on Mott Street, an old-school Chinese-American restaurant. I always ordered wonton soup and added a ton of Chinese mustard.

Sometimes, women came to meet us. One was a Polish woman called Zofia. She was very friendly. Zofia had a number tattooed on her forearm. My father explained quietly what it was. After lunch one weekend, we went uptown to Zofia's apartment. Dad said that he was going to install a ceiling fan in her bedroom. I watched TV and she and Dad went into the bedroom to put up the fan. When it was time to leave, I walked by the bedroom door and glanced in. There was no fan. When I mentioned this to my dad, he looked at me and said nothing.

The holidays weren't the same after Dad left. Mom started seeing a Puerto Rican woman with a nose ring and a fade. Her name was Wilma. I was fine with my mother dating a woman, but I didn't particularly like Wilma. She always needed money and she went with Richie to score drugs. I suffered through a few holidays with Mom and Wilma, but after Richie was murdered, I opted out altogether.

As soon as I got the job at the bagel store, I started to work every Thanksgiving. I've worked most holidays since then. If I'm not working, I spend them with Mike Sullivan, my friend from my Harlem days and one of the original members of the Group Home. Mike is based in the Bronx now and we rarely work together, but we're still like brothers. We go on trips; we hike; I go to see Mike's plays. Mike started acting again a few years ago and he's in a fringe theater group. I gave up acting pretty soon after I became an EMT. I did a couple of auditions and then it fizzled out. Though in a way, I perform every day: playing the wise medic, putting on a reassuring show for the families, sharing patients' stories and their pain.

Mike hates Christmas. He grew up in the closet with a police-chief dad and a domineering mom. There wasn't a lot of communication, and Mike felt the holidays were a charade. On Christmas, if Mike and I are together, we go to Katz's Deli and get pastrami sandwiches, then we cross East Houston to the little park on the north side and smoke cigars. It's our tradition. It gives meaning to a day that we both dread.

Once or twice, we've worked a holiday together. I convinced Mike to come to Brooklyn to work New Year's Eve in 2006. We caught the first shooting of 2007; it was in East New York, a neighborhood in

Brooklyn. The patient was a young Black guy who said he had shot himself in the hand drawing his gun on another man. Idiots like that guarantee that people like me will always be employed.

Mike and I also transported a couple who had been in a car accident to a hospital on Atlantic Avenue. The emergency department was chaos. There was a guy who had cut open the sole of his foot. He sat with his foot bleeding into a bucket. Then he got up and walked around, trailing blood everywhere.

"This is medieval!" Mike cried. "I wanna go back to the Bronx!"

The Bronx is the New York emergency service's busiest and toughest borough. It's hard to shock a medic who works there. But I had done it. Another proud moment for Brooklyn.

Thanksgiving 2019, we had a good crowd at Station 40, about twenty in all. Some of the people I was closest with at Station 40 were on duty. Angie was there, as was Albert "Birdman" Brigandi, who was cheap as they come but would drop forty thousand to buy a homing pigeon without blinking. And Alfonso "Bones" Buoninfante. (Like members of the Mafia, most of us have nicknames.) Bones had twenty years on the job and was an incredibly competent EMT. He spoke English and Brooklyn Italian and was very loquacious. He also had the whole pay-scale and pension system in his head, so he schooled us on pension plans.

Also at Thanksgiving that year was James "Jimmy Mac" McGuire, a former Wall Street trader with a wide forehead and a sweet smile. Jimmy lost his job in the Great Recession and became a paramedic. Very dedicated. He was one of Angie's partners on the ambulance. He usually drove; Angie had moved to Brooklyn from the Bronx earlier that year and was still shaky on the geography of the borough. Jimmy was always the last to sit down to eat and the first to clear the table.

Alex Loutsky was there too. He was a lieutenant paramedic and we usually worked the same tour, one on the road and one in the station. Alex was the first 911 responder to radio Emergency Dispatch with the news that a plane had hit the World Trade Center. He nearly suffocated in the dust and smoke after the first tower fell.

For our Thanksgiving feast, we cooked a twenty-six-pound turkey. I used a syringe to inject drippings into the breast. Because my arm was still weak, I had to ask an EMT to lift the turkey from the oven so I could baste it.

I was beginning to realize how badly my injury was handicapping me and it bothered me. EMS is a strenuous business. You're constantly lugging human beings and heavy gear. I took pride in being able to pull my weight—literally. At six foot one, I weighed about two hundred and fifty-five pounds, but now I couldn't lift a turkey.

Still, the meal was fun. Everyone brought a dish: mac and cheese, brussels sprouts with pancetta, garlic mashed potatoes. And a horrible string-bean salad. Every year, somebody brought a salad of canned beans and Italian dressing. Nobody ate it. Nobody owned up to bringing it. I had a list of suspects, but I won't share it here.

"Turkey's great, Lou," one of the EMTs said. (*Lou* is short for *lieutenant*.)

The table fell quiet. Everyone was eating. I was happy. I found few things more satisfying than cooking for people who enjoy my food.

Kelly Quirke broke the silence. Kelly was an EMT. Her dad was a firefighter and Kelly ate up all things firefighter—she even had a purse made from a firefighter's coat. "We got Patricia this morning," she said. "That woman is batshit crazy."

Patricia was one of our regulars, the people we called frequent fliers because we picked them up so often. We knew the regulars' Social Security numbers; we knew their birthdays; we knew if they had allergies. If they had an address, we knew that too.

Patricia called 911 several times a week. She lived in a brick palace in Borough Park. The house had a double staircase leading to the front door and balconies. It had hedges outside that were pruned into spirals. Patricia had no physical issue that we'd ever been able to find, but she had crippling anxiety. She didn't work. She didn't clean. She didn't cook. She was wealthy enough to have a housekeeper. Her kids went to high school. So Patricia sat in bed, rattled with fear. Every ache. Every pain. Every tiny discomfort, Patricia thought she was dying. So she called 911. Sometimes more than once a day. If her kids were there, they opened the front door and stood to the side. They looked mortified. They knew there was nothing wrong with their mother.

That morning, Patricia had said she couldn't breathe. But the crew had checked her vitals and they were perfect.

"Same old, same old," said Kelly.

"Did I tell you guys about the suicide that I had down near Prospect Park?" I asked.

"Suicide?" said Birdman. "I didn't hear that one."

"Couple of days ago," I said. "Guy in his eighties. He blew his brains out in the front yard." The man's brains were splattered all over the stoop of the house next door. Blood and lumps of jelly-like matter were stuck to the brownstone. It looked like raw hamburger. "The guy was sitting in a metal lawn chair with a blanket across his knees. Shot himself in the temple with a revolver. He still had the gun in his hand."

"Why'd he do it?" Kelly said.

"Cop at the scene said that his wife had died a week or so ago. I guess he decided that it was his time."

I had found the scene strangely peaceful. The man had lived a long life, and he'd gone out on his own terms. He'd apparently been devoted to his wife. The idea of having someone who meant that much to you—and of meaning that much to someone—made me envious. Luckily the bullet he'd used to kill himself hadn't hit any of the neighbors.

I got up to fetch myself some more food. This was the cue for somebody to go one better than me, try to outdo my brains-on-the-stoop story. But no one did. We ate dessert. For a day, I was the reigning champion.

It didn't last. The next afternoon, Kenny Craig upstaged me big-time.

Kenny was an awesome EMT. Good-looking. In his late twenties. At the time, Kenny had been on the job for a couple of years, but he was already wiser than some veterans. I'd clone Kenny if it were possible. A department full of Kennys—that's my dream.

The day after Thanksgiving, Kenny was assigned to a call for an emotionally disturbed person, an EDP, a few blocks from the station. An EDP is somebody who is behaving in a way that's irrational or bizarre and could be dangerous. The person might be mentally ill or in a state of severe crisis or depressed. We get calls for EDPs all the time.

Kenny went into the house of a Chinese family. They showed him into a bedroom. He was expecting to find a person in some sort of distress. But instead of an EDP, he saw a guy lying on the bed. Still as a statue. Blanket over his face. For a second, Kenny thought he was sleeping. He approached the patient and pulled back the blanket.

"The guy was dead. Ice cold," Kenny said.

As Kenny spoke, he stood in the doorway of my office. He had dropped into the station to collect supplies. I nodded. "Go on," I said.

"Okay. It gets weirder," Kenny said. "The guy had a noose around his neck."

Kenny said he'd asked the family what had happened. A young woman explained in broken English that they had found the man hanging from a tree in the garden. He was the woman's father or uncle; it wasn't clear. The family had cut the man down and brought him inside. They put him in bed, pulled the covers over him. And they'd left the noose tied around his neck. It was a thick rope that had cut a deep groove in the man's skin.

Kenny examined the corpse. The man had no pulse. He wasn't breathing. He was dead. But the crew couldn't tell how long he'd been like this, so they started CPR just in case there was a chance they could revive him. They called a paramedic unit for backup.

There was nothing to be done. The family seemed unmoved. Kenny and his partner left the medics with the family and drove away.

"Okay, Kenny," I said. "That's totally nuts. You got me."

In emergency medicine, we like to outdo each other. It keeps us humble. It's quite a trip for a twenty-something to be given the keys to a $144,000 ambulance. And when you rescue people for a living, it's easy to get a big head and start to think you're a superhero.

In reality, we're a bunch of broken toys. A lot of people who work in EMS grew up in messed-up environments or suffered trauma as kids. According to one study, the rate of suicide in EMS is more than double the rate in the general population. That has a lot to do with the trauma they see every day. And the poor pay. But there's also the fact that a lot of EMS workers are damaged before they set foot in EMT school.

When an EMS worker is dismissive about a patient who's obese or has a drinking problem, I say, "Motherfucker, you're no better than they are. You drink. You're up to your ears in debt." And it's true. FDNY patients tend to come from marginalized communities, but so do the EMS workers who serve them. Most of our patients wind up in the ambulance because of chronic disease, domestic violence, shootings, or addiction—afflictions that the EMTs and paramedics have also experienced. We mirror our patients.

Of course, that's not true of everyone. There are people in EMS who come from perfectly functional backgrounds. Some join the profession after careers on Wall Street or in retail. They want to give back to society. Look at Jimmy McGuire, Joe Cengiz, Greg Hodge. There are recruits from affluent neighborhoods who know that there's another New York out there and want to experience it. For those people, EMS is like Narnia. You step out of the wardrobe and—whoa!—you're in Brownsville.

They don't all enjoy what they find, mind you. About a year into my time as an EMT in Harlem, a woman named Jenny joined my bus fresh out of the academy. She was in her forties and had worked for years in a financial job of some sort. She had short hair and glasses.

I told Jenny that the best way to learn was to jump straight in. Jenny said she was ready. So all day I buffed calls. We did twelve jobs in eight hours. At one point, we transported a stab victim to Harlem Hospital; his guts were bursting out of his abdomen like a cauliflower. Jenny had blood all over her arm. She looked a little queasy.

"Is it l-like this every day?" she stammered.

"It can be," I told her. I was pretty cocky.

The next day, Jenny quit.

Growing up with plates crashing against walls and close relatives dying prepared me for this job. It made me hypervigilant. I was always on the alert, always ready to spring. It also gave me empathy, an emotional map that I can look at with another person and say, "You've been there? Me too."

Take the Bedford Atlantic Armory shelter in Crown Heights. Men sleep there in huge dormitories. They pin their shoes to the floor with the legs of their beds so that nobody can make off with them. When I visit a homeless asthmatic or an EDP in the shelter, I will nod and say, "Bro, I feel you. I spent a night here myself."

Once, I was in the apartment of an elderly lady and noticed photos of two men in green prison uniforms. I figured they were her sons. I pointed to one of the photos. I recognized the building in the background.

"Is that Elmira?" I asked.

"Yes," she said. "Have you been there?"

"Sure have," I said.

Several times.

When I was eight years old, Mom got it into her head that I should go with her to visit my brother, Richie, in jail. We went to Columbus Circle in Manhattan at five a.m. and caught a bus to Elmira Correctional Facility. Elmira is a massive redbrick maximum-security prison in upstate New York, near the Finger Lakes. Richie was serving time there for armed robbery and aggravated assault.

Over the years, I visited Richie in two prisons. One was Elmira; the other was Fishkill Correctional Facility in Beacon, New York. I went to Richie's wedding there during his second jail stint. We all dressed up and filed into a room that was used as a chapel. Three prisoners carried in a tall crucifix for the ceremony. They hung it on the wall. When the wedding was over, they came and took the crucifix down.

On my first trip to Elmira, Mom and I sat near the rear of the bus. It was dark and quiet. The other passengers nodded off. My mom also slept. We wouldn't get to Elmira until about ten a.m. I was too wired to sleep, so I read *Mad* magazine.

We had been on the road for a while when a young Black woman came to the back of the bus to use the restroom, which was a row or two behind us. She was pretty. I guess she was in her twenties, but I was so young I probably couldn't gauge her age. She went into the restroom, but she didn't lock the door properly or maybe the lock was broken. The door kept banging with the movement of the bus. I turned to look. All of a sudden, the door swung open wide to reveal the woman crouching on top of the toilet. She had her panties around her ankles, and she was holding small, colored balloons.

The woman spread her vagina open with her fingers and inserted a balloon. My eyes nearly popped out of my head. I had never seen a woman's genitals. I had no idea they could be used to store things.

The woman caught me watching her. She smiled. Then she inserted another balloon. I kept looking away and looking back at her. I was fascinated.

When she was finished, she hopped down from the toilet and pulled up her underwear. She walked back to the front of the bus. As she passed me, she gave me a pat on the shoulder.

When Mom woke up, I told her what I had seen. She smiled. "Whoever that girl's visiting, she's just trying to keep them safe," she said.

At the prison, we sat with Richie. I asked him if he felt safe.

"Sure," he said. "I'm safe. I'm okay. Don't worry, Anthony."

I wondered what that meant.

On the bus ride home, I asked my mother, "Do you do what that woman was doing?"

"Do what?" Mom said.

"You know. What the lady was doing in the bathroom. Richie said he's safe. Does that mean that you do what she was doing?"

Mom laughed. "I don't do that, Anthony."

We sat in silence. I pulled back the gray curtain and looked out the window at the trees. Then Mom said, "When we get back, I'll show you what I do to take care of Richie."

A few days later, Mom took me to Union Street, between Fourth and Fifth Avenues. Union Street is in what real estate agents nowadays call North Slope. It's the fancy end of Park Slope. But it wasn't fancy then. Many of the brick and brownstone houses had their windows boarded up.

Mom stopped at a doorway covered in peeling green paint. She knocked. A guy opened the door. We went inside. The man gave Mom some little bags. They contained a whitish powder. Mom gave the guy cash. Then we walked the sixteen blocks home to Thirteenth Street. It was like walking to a different world.

At home, Mom put the bags on the dining table. Mom did everything at that table. She sat there to pay the bills every month—she licked the stamps, stuck them to the envelopes, then slid the envelopes under her buttocks to press the stamps down. (Years after this, she sat at the table with Wilma and came out to me. And she was sitting at the table when she learned that Richie was dead.)

Mom boiled some water in a pan on the stove. She got out several bars of Irish Spring soap. Each was wrapped in dark green paper with a clover leaf on it. Mom took a bar of soap with its paper wrapping and held it above the boiling water. She steamed open the wrapper. She slid the soap out. She did that again and again. Then she grabbed a potato peeler, sat down at the table, and used the scoop at the end to hollow out the bars of soap, one by one. She collected all the shavings carefully in a pile. She took the bags of powder and emptied them into the cavities in the soap. Then she packed the soap shavings on top of the powder. She smoothed the bars with sandpaper. She wrapped each soap in paper again and used a dab of glue to close it. Very meticulous.

"What are you doing?" I asked.

"I want your brother to be safe," said Mom. She explained that if she could get drugs to Richie, bad people in prison would leave him alone. She added, "If I don't do this, he will never make it in that place."

"Don't tell anyone about the soap or the man on Union Street," Mom said. I nodded.

"Nobody," she said.

"I won't, Mom."

Mom said, "I want you to remember all of this, Anthony. Keep it in your mind."

Mom always wanted me to learn. She taught me the alphabet when I was a baby. She read me stories every night. But taking me to see my brother in prison? Taking me with her to score drugs? Did she want me to see the lengths she'd go to in order to protect her children? The importance of studying and staying out of trouble? I'm still not sure.

Those experiences did do one thing for me. I was able to sit with that old lady with her photos of her incarcerated sons and tell her I had some idea of the pain that she'd gone through.

Sometimes I take empathy to an extreme. After my father died of liver failure, in 2012, I started to get panic attacks again. I had panic attacks as a kid, so I knew what they felt like, but I hadn't had them for a long time.

I was on the ambulance one day with a medic named Tim Bittar. We were called to a possible heart attack on Rogers Avenue in Crown Heights. I started to feel a tingling in my hands, and my brow was clammy. I was breathing fast. During a panic attack, you take rapid, shallow breaths and breathe out carbon dioxide too quickly. That alters the pH of your blood and leads to alkalosis. Alkalosis causes the blood vessels to constrict, reducing blood supply to the brain. You feel light-headed. Your lips get numb. You get cramping in your extremities.

If you keep breathing that way, your brain shuts you down and you pass out.

Tim asked me if I wanted to stay in the ambulance. "No, I'm good," I said.

In the elevator, I leaned against the wall and closed my eyes. I breathed slowly. When we reached the apartment, Tim took the lead. The patient described his symptoms. He felt tingling and numbness, he said. Difficulty catching his breath. He was anxious. He had just been diagnosed with HIV.

What I did next sounds ridiculous, but it seemed natural at the time. I walked over to the man and said, "Brother, I think you're having a panic attack. You're not going to believe this, but I'm having a panic attack too."

I sat down beside the man, and he clasped my hand. He asked me what was going on with me. I asked him what was going on with him. We breathed slowly. Tim and I ran an EKG on him, just to rule out a heart problem.

As we left, the man thanked me.

"I'm the one who should be thanking you," I said. "You talked me down."

The bump I got from the trip to Hong Kong and China didn't last. I quickly slumped again. I dreaded getting my arm fixed. It would mean missing weeks of work and recovering at home, by myself.

And my heart was wounded too. Just before Thanksgiving, the woman I was dating said that she wanted to take a break. Things had been going well before Joe died; she seemed to find me attractive and apparently enjoyed being with somebody who was affectionate. I was nuts about her. She was smart, funny. We'd lie around in bed on our days off. I have a tendency to hold on to women too tightly, but this time I tried to hold back a little. And it had been working.

After Joe passed, though, I became depressed and lost my sex drive. I'd had an awkward conversation with her. I'd told her that I still loved her but that I couldn't be physical. She was sweet about it and said it didn't matter and that she understood. But I imagine that she was a little confused.

When I returned from Hong Kong, I thought I had turned a corner. I told her I was feeling better. She seemed pleased. A few days later, though, I tried to kiss her and she backed away. She wanted "friend Anthony," not "boyfriend Anthony," she said.

I tried to be cool about her wanting to take a break. I said she could have as much time as she needed. But in my heart, I knew. Once a woman demotes you to friend status, you never make it back to being her boyfriend.

Joe's death had got me thinking. In a way, I'm glad that I was with him after he collapsed. I have the comfort of knowing that we did everything we could to save him, that we'd tried to help an old friend. Joe was a loner. Sociable but reserved. He didn't really hang out with anyone from work besides me and one other medic. Maybe fate intervened to have me work the day he got sick.

But Joe's death had rattled my confidence. His sister and brother-in-law were devastated. They thanked us again and again for all that we'd done. But I felt I had let them down. Joe had helped train me. With Joe as my lieutenant, I'd treated dozens of people with serious heart attacks. Some of them I had saved. But not Joe. I'd failed him.

The whole thing also felt like a warning. Joe had worked hard his whole life. He'd spent a quarter of a century in EMS and a decade or more driving a taxi. He'd thought he would spend his twilight years taking long walks and setting up a café in Turkey. And how long did he get? Four months? And then he died.

What happened to Joe could easily happen to me, I thought. Instead of kicking back and enjoying retirement, I could end up in a hospital bed in Brooklyn, taking my last breaths through a tube.

Anthony, I tell you to slow down, but you don't listen, Joe said in my head. *How about this: I'll tear your fucking biceps tendon. That'll slow you down.*

And it did. A little. Perhaps not in the way that Joe would have wanted—I fell behind in the classes I was taking at Brooklyn College in an attempt to finish my bachelor's degree (almost twenty years in the making). I needed twenty-seven more credits, but after I hurt my arm and missed some classes, I decided to drop out for the semester.

Still, I could manage most things. So I ignored Joe's warning again. Instead of getting the surgery as quickly as possible, I stuck with plans to visit Australia and New Zealand for a month with Angie. I couldn't miss it. Travel is everything to me. When I'm not on a trip, I'm planning a trip or talking about a trip I've just taken. I'd visited nearly ninety countries over the previous twenty years, but I'd never been as far as Australia and New Zealand. I'd get my arm fixed when I got back, I thought. There would be time.

I kept telling myself, *Anthony, December 27, you're going to be on a plane. You just gotta get there. Australia. New Zealand. You're gonna complete the circuit.* "Mom! Dad! Look at me," *you'll say.* "Look at what I did! Despite all the shit that happened, I made it around the world."

DECEMBER 2019

Emergency medicine has strange rhythms. One minute, you're idling in an ambulance playing Candy Crush or reading or catching up on medical protocols. The next, you're screeching toward an asthmatic whose airways have constricted to the point of suffocation or a woman who is giving birth on the floor of the A train. As EMTs and medics, we have no control. We don't make things happen. We wait for them to happen to other people. Then we respond. Our puppet master is the radio. It chirps and crackles day and night, a stream of codes. It's a ticker of South Brooklyn sickness and injury.

"Conditions Four-Three, you're going to West Eighth Street and Bay Parkway for the trauma. You're assisting Thirty-Three Adam. Conditions Four-Three."

Conditions Four-Three is the call sign of the lieutenant at Station 43. Thirty-Three Adam is an ambulance crew.

"Conditions Four-Three, sixty-three. Helping Thirty-Three Adam. Give us a ten-twelve when they are eighty-four. Thank you."

Sixty-three means they are on their way. *Eighty-four* means they are on scene.

"Thirty-Three Adam, when you get on scene, please give me a ten-twelve for Conditions . . . Four-Two Boy, Sixty-Fifth Street and Ridge Boulevard for the altered mental. Four-Two Boy . . . Four-Zero Adam, are you still sixty-three? Four-Zero Adam."

"Still sixty-three. Two minutes out."

The Dispatch radio is the white noise of EMS. For me, it's like listening to the ocean. And when the dispatcher calls my unit, it's like a foghorn in my ear. I jump to it. Even if I'm asleep. Fully reclined, snoring a little. When my call sign comes over the air, I reach for the radio and reply before I've even opened my eyes. In an instant, I have the keys in the ignition and then I'm flying through the streets. (I knew an EMT whose wife woke him up by leaning close to his ear and murmuring his call sign. "Three-Two Adam," the wife would say. A second later, her husband was awake.)

There is one time when you can count on hearing your call sign: When you've just bought hot food. You climb into the ambulance, your stomach rumbling, holding a fried-egg sandwich on a toasted bagel or an order of *tacos de lengua*. And—bang!—the fickle gods of EMS drop a call into your lap.

One afternoon a few days before Christmas, the EMS gods paid me a visit. I was working on the road. It was a slow day. I'd had only two calls that morning: a man who called an ambulance so the crew would carry him up the stairs of his apartment building ("Sorry, brother, we don't do carry-ups," I'd told him) and a drunk who refused to let us bring him to the ED so he could get a banana bag (an IV infusion of electrolytes and vitamins; I convinced him to go). Between calls, I texted Sara Lupin—the lieutenant paramedic who met me at Maimonides the day that Joe fell sick—about watering my plants while I was in Australia and New Zealand. Sara's another member of the Group Home. Unless she's traveling with me, Sara always takes care of my plants. She loves plants and has a lot of them, so I figure she won't kill mine.

I was hungry and gloomy over Joe. I decided to get lunch and take it to my favorite spot, a derelict pier in Sunset Park. A family of Canada geese live there. When it's quiet on the road, I swing by to check on them.

I stopped at a Mexican food truck a few blocks from Station 40, bought tacos and a lemonade, and drove down to the water.

• • •

As I was parking on the waterfront, a middle-aged man driving a semi-trailer across the Verrazzano-Narrows Bridge passed out at the wheel and crashed his truck. The man's name was Daniel.

Daniel was on his way to Staten Island—the bridge connects the island to Brooklyn—when he had a heart attack. His heart was deprived of oxygen and went haywire. It produced erratic electrical impulses that did not allow it to beat properly. The ventricles—the lower heart chambers that pump blood around the body—quivered instead of pumping, an irregular rhythm called ventricular fibrillation.

Once Daniel's heart stopped pumping sufficient blood to his brain, his brain function became impaired. Maybe he gasped periodically as if he were trying to get more air, something called agonal breathing. It's a brain-stem reflex that happens when the organs aren't getting enough oxygen. Eventually, the medulla oblongata, the part of Daniel's brain stem that controlled involuntary respiration, shut down.

Daniel ceased breathing. Clinically speaking, he was dead.

Hours before he passed out, Daniel probably felt a bit of soreness in his left arm. Fatigue. But long-distance truckers are always sleep-deprived. Daniel most likely shrugged it off, maybe stopped in a gas station and bought himself an extra cup of coffee. Maybe he noticed that it took a little extra effort to climb back into the truck and told himself it was time to get a checkup. I will never know.

By the time Daniel drove into Brooklyn, he must have been feeling very uncomfortable. Sweating. Finding it hard to get a good breath. And then the pain in his chest must have become overwhelming; he probably tried to gulp air in long gasps. Before he lost consciousness, Daniel might have pumped the brakes of his truck. The heavy traffic on the bridge would have meant that he was moving slowly, so he didn't go careening off the edge of the bridge or smash into a column of cars. He just flopped over the steering wheel, and his eighty-foot semi veered right and tipped over. It lay on its side across three lanes like a great creature brought down by a bullet. Daniel dangled, lifeless, in the driver's seat, his seat belt holding him in place.

. . .

The waterfront where I eat my lunch is on the edge of a maze of brick warehouses: garment factories, film-production studios, lumberyards, a halal store where I sometimes buy live chickens. (I started going there a few years back because I wanted to reconnect with the food that I eat. I wasn't going to become a vegetarian like the Buddha, but I still wanted to honor the animal and understand its sacrifice. The guys in the store would hand me a chicken and I'd wring its neck right there in the shop.)

The area was once an industrial hub, one of the biggest in the United States. Until a few decades ago, there were piers all the way up the waterfront, from Sunset Park to the Gowanus Canal and Red Hook. You can still see the iron railroad tracks peeking through the asphalt. I love the neighborhood. It reminds me of my dad. He worked on the piers until the late 1980s, when they moved the port to New Jersey, on the other side of the harbor. Dad was forced to follow.

It was near the waterfront that I received my first lesson in labor relations. I was eight or nine. The Seafarers International Union was on strike because the shipping company Dad worked for wanted to cut one of their vacation checks ($5,000 bonuses that were given four times a year to coincide roughly with vacations). Dad took me down to the picket line. There were thousands of strikers stretched along five blocks on Third Avenue.

Dad explained to me that they were fighting the cuts because they didn't trust the bosses to invest that money in the company. "They want to keep it for themselves," he said. "Once you give an inch to these people, you never get it back."

The strikers dug in their heels and won.

The incident lit a little flame in me that got bigger over the years. At the bagel store, I argued that the staff should get a lunch break so we could sit and eat. We wound up getting fifteen minutes—better than nothing. At a shoe store I worked at, I fought to have the sales staff pool their commissions so the people working the quieter shifts didn't get the shit end of the stick. In 2006, I became a union delegate for Local 2507, the EMTs and paramedics union at Station 38, and in 2018, I became vice president of the EMS officers' union, Local 3621.

I pulled up at the water's edge and turned off the engine. The geese often shelter beneath the pier, between pilings covered in dark green weeds. Next to the pier is a depot that belongs to the Department of Sanitation. There are lines of garbage trucks and a huge, collapsing shed where the department stores salt for the winter. It's pretty bleak. But it's quiet and the air has a briny smell.

I spied two of the Canada geese. I first saw them there a few years ago, and they always seem to be in the same place, so perhaps they don't migrate. Permanent Canadian immigrants. After I saw them, I began stopping at the waterfront whenever I could. Lunchtime, after work. My tracker friend Zak in Montana told me that to get in among wildlife, you have to remain very still. Become part of the scenery. So I turned off the engine of my truck. Left the radio on. Watched the birds.

The geese always waddled by me on the concrete, past the sanitation trucks and then back. I tried not to move. For half an hour, I felt as if I were outside my own head. It was peaceful. I tend to keep myself very busy, always doing a dozen things, always on the move—job, union, travel, friends; Twitter, Facebook, Instagram, texts. So I try to find moments to be still.

Practicing Buddhism helps in that respect. I meditate every day. I kneel in the corner of the bedroom in front of the altar. There's a small statue of the Buddha over which I've draped a gold necklace that belonged to my father and a *mala*—a string of prayer beads—that Richie's former wife, Holly, gave me. I focus on my breathing. Nostrils, lungs, abdomen. In. Out.

When I lose myself, I sit for hours. But a lot of days, I can't still my mind. I'm resentful or angry. So I sit for two minutes and then I'm done.

· · ·

A few weeks after I first encountered the geese, I started to bring them seeds, nuts. I scattered the food near me. There was one goose whose white chest-feathers were shaped like an off-center V. He and his mate edged closer. I offered them food from my hand. I had this idea of being a goose whisperer, of being able to communicate with the animal kingdom, of being like David Attenborough, standing in the Kalahari Desert with a meerkat on his shoulder. The male goose often came within about three feet of me, then backed away. Then one day, the bird came right up to me and took a piece of lettuce from my hand. I nearly jumped for joy.

In the spring of 2019, the pair had goslings. The parents continued to approach me, but they kept the babies at a distance. It was touching to see how protective they were of their young. The goslings grew bigger. Over the course of a few weeks, they started taking food from me. I felt like part of their family.

We always had animals in the house when I was a kid. Richie had turtles. A snake. When we took family trips upstate, he and I would hunt under rocks for spiders and garter snakes. In Brooklyn, we had a raccoon called Bandit and a monkey. I have no idea whether it was legal to keep monkeys or raccoons as pets in New York in those days. It isn't now. Either way, it was the 1980s, and nobody cared.

We also had a white poodle named Peaches. Mom thought I should have a pet to grow up with. She told me that she would have liked for me to have a little brother or sister, but she'd had a miscarriage after she had me. So instead of a new sibling, I got Peaches. Mom would take her to be groomed and have her nails painted pink.

When Richie died, we inherited his dog, Cujo. Cujo was a beautiful chow chow with a thick bronze coat and a halo of fur around his head. Richie took good care of him. He said that he'd gotten Cujo from a friend who owed him money. The friend didn't have the money, so he gave Richie the dog instead. It made sense.

But after Richie died, a friend told me how he'd really gotten Cujo: Richie and the friend had burgled a house on Staten Island. Cujo was in the house. Cujo was friendly. They took cash and jewelry and whatever else they wanted. The friend went out to the car to wait for Richie. Richie appeared with a bag over one shoulder and the dog under his arm. He stole a family's dog. That was Richie for you.

Making off with a family's pet wasn't the only line that Richie crossed. He stole my parents' television. He stole my baseball cards, including a Rickey Henderson and a Don Mattingly rookie card—priceless for a kid like me.

It was as if Richie thought the rules didn't apply to him. But even gangland has rules. And Richie broke those too. That was his undoing.

Richie went missing in May 1993, about two weeks after my sixteenth birthday. He was back from Fishkill on parole, and he was living in the apartment in the top of my mom's house. He and Holly were separated by then, and Holly was living in Staten Island. Little Anthony bounced between Holly and his grandmothers and Richie. Richie had a new girlfriend, Diane, who was very into him. She tried, without success, to straighten him out.

Richie had to be home at my mom's by nine p.m. as part of his parole agreement. When he didn't show one night, Mom tried to page him. Yvonne came in from Staten Island and the two of them drove around Brooklyn searching for Richie. Mom called the police. She called the morgue. She spent all night sitting at the table in the dining room. In the morning, I heard her making calls again. And then I heard her scream.

The police had found Richie's body rolled in a carpet. Apparently, they discovered him by chance. They had been called to a domestic dispute in a building in Park Slope that was next to the one where Richie had been murdered, but they'd gone into the wrong building. When they entered, Richie's murderer—a neighborhood guy named Strike—was coming down the stairs that led to the front door, dragging the carpet with Richie inside it.

In the spring before he died, Richie came home with a duffel bag full of weed. He showed it to me. He asked if I knew anyone who could sell it. I did. I had a couple of friends up the block. They packaged the weed into nickel bags and sold it.

A few weeks later, I found Richie standing in the dark in his apartment, peering out the window. "You see them?" he said.

I looked.

"Anthony, do you see them?"

"I don't see anyone, Richie," I said.

"They're after me, Ant," Richie said. "They're following me."

"Okay, Richie. Let's come away from the window," I said. "Maybe they'll leave."

We sat on the couch. I thought Richie was imagining things, but I played along—a skill I'd use in the ambulance in the years to come.

Richie didn't tell me, but it turned out that he had stolen the weed—along with cash and other drugs—from a guy linked to a big crime family. That's what Strike—a hoodlum whose real name was Alvin Aponte who hung out with Richie sometimes—told the police. Richie had broken into the guy's house and tied up a member of the household, Strike said. Tying the guy up crossed a line. So the mobster offered Strike ten grand to kill Richie, and Strike shot Richie in the temple.

After Mom hung up the phone, she put her head in her hands and wailed. I tried to put my arm around her, but she pushed me away.

The house filled with people. Yvonne. Kathy. Detectives, neighbors.

I couldn't bear to be around them, so I invited some friends to go to Yankee Stadium with me. I had a hundred bucks that Richie had given me for my birthday. I bought all of them seats in the bleachers. I bought hot dogs.

Jim Abbott pitched for the Yankees that night. Abbott was born without a right hand, but he was so skilled, you wouldn't know that he was playing one-handed. The Orioles beat the Yankees, eight to six. But it didn't matter. I just needed an escape.

When we paid our respects to Richie in the funeral home, I thought about a photo some detectives had shown me years earlier while they were investigating a murder on our street. The photo was of a woman who was killed in the stairwell of the building that my godmother, Kathy, took care of. She had been shot in the temple and she had what's called an eight-ball injury. That's when the eye fills with black-red blood and bulges like a pool ball.

Was Richie's eye like that after he was shot? I wondered.

I looked at Richie's temple. The mortician had plugged the hole with some kind of putty and smoothed wax over it. He'd done a very good job. But I couldn't stop thinking about the woman's black swollen eye.

Mom had Richie buried in a steel casket. It was a beautiful midnight blue lined with light blue satin. They lowered the casket into a stone tomb. Then they dropped a huge slab of stone across the top. Before they buried Richie, Mom had put a bag of heroin in his pocket. It was the only thing that made him happy, she said.

During the burial, Mom, Dad, Yvonne, Holly, and the rest of the extended family stood on one side of the grave. Richie's son, Anthony, stood between Holly and Yvonne. I stood on the other side, near the pastor and the grave diggers. I looked at my family from the other side of the hole in the ground. I didn't want to stand with them.

Sitting by the water in the command car with my lunch, I watched to see if any more geese appeared. I opened the Styrofoam taco container. I squeezed a wedge of lime over the meat and dribbled it with green sauce, then arranged the slices of radish inside the tacos. Perfect.

The EMS gods must have been laughing, though. I had barely taken a bite when the radio hissed.

"Conditions Four-O. Verrazzano Bridge, Staten Island–bound. MVA with injuries."

Every 911 call is assigned a call type. For example, *diff breather* means someone who is having difficulty breathing, maybe due to asthma or an allergic reaction. *MVA* is shorthand for *motor vehicle accident.*

As well as coming over the radio, the call appears on a screen mounted on the vehicle's dashboard. We can see what's going on in the field and send messages by hitting buttons at the bottom of the screen. We hit the button marked 98 to signal that we are clear of our last call and available for the next.

I reached for the radio handset. "Conditions Four-O. Sixty-three," I said. *I'm on my way.*

I sighed. I placed the taco container on the passenger seat. Put the truck in gear. Hit the siren.

Six minutes. If you go into cardiac arrest—your heart stops pumping, you stop breathing, you lose consciousness—that's how long we have to reach you. Clinical death occurs when the heart stops beating, but biological death occurs about six minutes later. That's when brain damage begins. Within six minutes, you need someone—bystander, medic, firefighter—to find you and start cardiopulmonary resuscitation.

Even then, your odds of survival are not good. Less than 10 percent of Americans who suffer a cardiac arrest outside a hospital setting live long enough to be admitted to the hospital, treated, and discharged.

And CPR is not a pretty business. It's not how it looks on television. The rescuer compresses the patient's chest so hard that the ribs can tear away from the sternum. There are cracking and popping sounds. And it's exhausting. If you have enough people on hand, you switch rescuers every two minutes.

Still, working on a cardiac patient with a group of experienced medics is a beautiful thing. There's very little talking. Everyone is incredibly focused. Everyone knows their role. It's like the universe is flowing through your hands. I put everything I have into CPR. "Like they owe you money," I tell the medics. "Pump like they owe you money."

And if you do get a pulse back, the high is unbeatable. Emergency medical workers are prone to addiction. We need our hit of dopamine, and this is our fix: The adrenaline of the call. The exertion of CPR. And the bolt of elation when you press your fingers to the neck of a lifeless person and feel the sudden thud of their heart.

A few days before Daniel's accident, I received a Christmas card from a man in Pennsylvania named Darren. As I read the card, I felt my heart swell.

Eleven years and forever grateful, Darren wrote. He wished me the best for 2020.

In 2008, Darren had been stocking shelves at a Family Dollar store on Fulton Street in Brooklyn. He sat down to rest for a minute. Then he passed out. I was working that day with Brendan Ryan, a new medic straight out of the academy; I'd picked him because I heard that he liked to get down.

When we walked into the store, Darren was lying in an aisle lined with boxes of cereal. He had his eyes open, but he wasn't breathing, and he had no pulse. I started CPR. Brendan took out the Lifepak—the brand of defibrillator that we carried at the time—and stuck pads on Darren's chest. The machine indicated ventricular fibrillation. Darren was in cardiac arrest.

When a patient is in cardiac arrest—that is, without a heartbeat—medical responders want to see one of two rhythms on the monitor: ventricular fibrillation (V-fib) or ventricular tachycardia (V-tach). Both rhythms are caused by an electrical problem. Both can be fixed—much of the time—with electrical current. We use a defibrillator to deliver a controlled electric shock to the heart, roughly enough electricity to light a 100-watt bulb for a few seconds. The patient rides the lightning.

In ventricular fibrillation, the heart quivers ineffectively, which was what Daniel's heart was doing. On a monitor, the rhythm presents as a shallow zigzag line. In ventricular tachycardia, the ventricles pump much too quickly. Instead of, say, sixty beats a minute, the heart beats one hundred and fifty times a minute or more, much too fast to pump blood efficiently. On the monitor, the rhythm produces a series of steep spikes.

What medics don't want to see is pulseless electrical activity, PEA. That means that the heart is still emitting electrical impulses, but the muscle isn't responding. It's like when you turn the key in the ignition of a car and nothing happens. The lights come on, but the engine doesn't crank. PEA is not a rhythm we can shock. We have to perform CPR to keep the blood flowing and race the patient to the emergency department. Physicians will either operate or use drugs to try to fix the problem that caused the heart to break down.

We shocked Darren and intubated him. We shocked him again. When we arrived at the hospital, he was biting the breathing tube. (That's a good thing—it means the patient is alive and conscious.)

That year, the fire department invited Darren to a brunch that we host for the people we save. We call it the Second Chance Brunch. I've gone two or three times. The brunch is funded by the family of a wealthy businessman named Jack Pintchik. Pintchik's family owns a lot of paint stores. In 1980, Jack was visiting a new store in downtown Brooklyn when he had a heart attack and went into cardiac arrest. Two paramedics revived him.

The FDNY sends out invitations, picks up the former patients, and brings them to the function on Randall's Island. We all sit at long tables with plastic cloths in the cafeteria of the FDNY's training academy. EMTs, firefighters, and medics are on one side; the guests are on the other. It's awkward as hell. But you see all these people who were clinically dead and got a second shot.

At the brunch, Darren walked over to me and Brendan. He hugged us both. He had tears in his eyes. Then a little girl peeped out from behind his legs. She was knee-high to a duck. Kindergartner, I would guess.

"Thank you for saving my daddy," she said.

I blinked hard a few times and knelt down to meet her eye.

"You're welcome," I said. "You hungry?"

At the same brunch, I met a seventy-two-year-old woman whom the medics had shocked twelve times. Twelve! Five would be a high number. I remembered the woman's case because I'd bumped into the medics in the emergency department just after they saved her. I said hello to the old lady and the medics. We crowded together for a photograph. She was very sweet, smiling at everyone.

A few months after the brunch, I answered a call at an apartment in Crown Heights. An elderly woman sat inside on the couch. She wore a brown wig. I recognized her immediately. The lady from the brunch!

The old woman said she had chest pain. I asked her if she was taking medication. When did you last eat or drink? I asked. No meds, said Grandma. I told her that I remembered her, that my friends had saved her. Oh yes, the old lady said. Her face lit up. Very nice people, she said.

What was she doing when she began to feel unwell? I asked. She shrugged. She pointed to a crack pipe that lay on the coffee table.

"I was smoking that," she said.

Not everyone makes the most of a second chance.

More often than not, we EMTs and paramedics don't know what happens to our patients. We are in and out of their lives in forty-five minutes. We don't know if the MVA victim kept his leg or if the elderly man died from sepsis or if the young teenager gave birth to a healthy baby. Sometimes a nurse or a doctor updates us. And every now and then, we get a letter from a patient like Darren.

Or from Adam's mom. Every February since 2018, Angie has received a greeting card from Rosario, the mother of this young boy, Adam. They live in the Bronx. When Rosario went into labor in 2017, Adam was in a breech presentation, meaning that his feet would be delivered first, not his head. Adam's dad called 911. Rosario climbed into the bathtub in her tiny bathroom in University Heights.

When Angie reached the scene, Rosario's husband and young daughter were in the living room. Four firefighters huddled outside the bathroom doorway. An EMT stood on the toilet, administering oxygen. Another EMT, clearly panicking, leaned over the edge of the bath.

Angie pushed past the firefighters and EMTs and climbed into the tub. Rosario was Latina, in her twenties, petite. Angie's Dominican. She spoke to Rosario in rapid Spanish. I understand a bit of Spanish, but I don't understand Angie's. She sounds like running water. As Angie spoke to Rosario, she felt the umbilical cord with her fingertips. There was no pulse.

The baby's heart had stopped beating.

Angie can be very stern when she needs to be. (When we were on a job in the Bronx once, a patient's mother became hysterical. We'd just sent the patient off in an ambulance, and the woman was wailing in the middle of the street. We kept trying to get her to sit in our ambulance, but she wouldn't stop screaming. "Ma'am. Please," I said. "We need you to get into the ambulance." The woman ignored me. Angie walked up to the woman and snapped her fingers in her face three times. "Get into the fucking ambulance," she said. "We are not doing this here." The woman looked at her in amazement and then climbed right in.)

Angie looked at Rosario lying in the bathtub with her lifeless baby's leg sticking out of the birth canal. "You need to push this baby out," Angie said. *"Right now."*

Rosario took a huge breath and pushed. The baby slid out, limp and pale. His face was blue. Angie climbed out of the bathtub, wrapped him in a sheet, and cradled him in the crook of her left arm. She pumped his chest with two fingers, then put a bag-valve mask over his face and squeezed air into his lungs. Her partner was in the ambulance, calculating doses of medication to give to the baby. Angie ran down the stairs to the ambulance, alternately squeezing the bag and pumping the tiny chest. A firefighter jumped into the driver's seat. Angie and her partner rode in the back.

They drove like the wind to St. Barnabas Hospital, a mile and a half away. Angie pumped the baby's chest with two fingers. Her partner squeezed puffs of air into his lungs. Squeezing, pressing, counting, squeezing, pressing, counting, they ran through the doors of the emergency department and over to the team of physicians and nurses who were waiting with the crash cart (a cabinet on wheels that contains tools and medications for treating cardiac arrest). As Angie lowered Adam onto the gurney, she felt a tiny beat. Then another. And then the faint whoosh of blood running through the baby's vessels.

Angie's not an emotional person. She grew up in the Bronx with a needy mother who'd been abused as a child, a brother who ended up in jail, and another brother who was killed in a motorcycle accident. Her father was a lovely man and very supportive, but Angie learned early on that there was little to be gained by talking about your feelings. To survive in her neighborhood, she had to be tough.

But when Angie felt the life returning to that baby's body, she dissolved into tears.

Sometimes, a patient gets in touch years later. Thanks to Facebook, I am in contact with a couple named Nick and Audrey. Nick is a nurse, and Audrey restores stained glass. They live in Ohio with their two young kids. But Nick and Audrey lived in Brooklyn when they were in their late twenties, and that's when I treated Nick.

Nick was slim and in good shape. He worked as an administrative assistant for a corporate employee-volunteer program and ran half-marathons, and he had recently started dating Audrey. On March 18, 2008, Nick woke up with terrible chest pain. He threw up. His vision came and went. He phoned Audrey for help, and as he spoke to her, his arm became numb, and he found it hard to move his hand. Audrey rushed over to his apartment. She gave him water and crackers. She looked up Nick's symptoms on WebMD, and they decided he had indigestion. Payback for a St. Patrick's Day blowout the day before. But the pain in Nick's chest became unbearable and he began to cough up pink sputum.

When my partner and I arrived at Nick's apartment building on Eastern Parkway, he was outside in his coat, hunched over. An EMT crew was with him.

Nick described the pain in his chest as a tearing sensation. (He told me years later that it was like being stabbed with a fourteen-inch Wüsthof knife.) The pain radiated toward his back, he said. My partner went to grab some nitroglycerine, which we use to treat angina—chest pain that is caused by insufficient blood flow to the heart. Nitro is a vasodilator, meaning it opens up the vessels to increase blood flow.

"Wait a minute," I said. I was thinking of a woman I'd treated in Coney Island a few years earlier. Like Nick, she was youngish. Like Nick, she had a tearing pain in her chest that radiated to her back. Like Nick, she had different blood pressure measurements in each arm; the reading from her right arm was 220/160; the left arm was 120/80. And like Nick's, her sputum was pink.

The woman had an aortic dissection. She was dead within the hour.

An aortic dissection often starts as a weak area in the aorta, the large vessel that feeds blood from your heart to the rest of your body. The pressure of your blood in the vessel can damage the tissue and lead to a tear between the layers of the aorta. This is called a dissection. It's incredibly painful. If blood escapes through the tear and into the lungs, you cough up bloody sputum. If the wall of the aorta ruptures—that is, if it gives way completely—you'll bleed out internally.

As we rushed the woman to Coney Island Hospital, she turned to me and said that the pain had gone. I yelled to my partner through the boot—the opening between the back of the ambulance and the cab—"Go! Go!"

But it was too late. The patient coded, and we couldn't bring her back. Her chest cavity had filled with blood.

As I remembered my ambulance ride with that woman, I feared for Nick. There was a significant chance he would die.

"Okay, Nick," I said. I patted his arm. "It's okay. We're going to get you to the hospital."

When you have a patient with an aortic dissection, you want to keep his blood pressure down. You want to minimize the strain on the vessel and get him to a surgeon. I told the EMTs to alert the staff at Methodist Hospital in Park Slope. It's one of two hospitals in Brooklyn that have a cardiothoracic center. We inserted an IV into Nick's arm so we could give him fluids if his blood pressure suddenly dropped.

The surgical team at Methodist met us downstairs and swept Nick inside. The surgeons replaced his torn aortic valve with a titanium valve and inserted an endovascular stent graft—a piece of synthetic tubing—in the damaged section of the aorta. When Nick woke up, the nurses told him it was a miracle that he had survived.

"Apparently, you have something left to do on this earth," they said.

Nick recovered. The mechanical valve in his heart beat so loudly at first that he joked he was the Tin Man. Nick began speaking at events organized by the American Heart Association, but he wanted to do more. In 2012, he started training to become a nurse. He specializes in cardiac care, and since 2017, he has worked in the cardiac telemetry unit of Atrium Medical Center in Middletown, Ohio. Sometimes, to encourage patients, he tells them about the day he nearly died. It still gives him goose bumps. He inspired one patient to become a nurse too. People talk about the butterfly effect, how small things can lead to big changes. I often think that kind of talk is bullshit. But then I meet someone like Nick, and I wonder.

Nick is gentle and has a wiry build. He meditates every day. He's not allowed to run anymore, so he lifts weights instead. At night, after a long shift on the cardiac floor, he lies down with his children and reads to them. The kids rest their heads on Nick's chest. They listen to the click of his titanium valve.

"Daddy," they say, "we can hear your heart."

. . .

It's a quick sprint from the waterfront in Sunset Park to the Verrazzano Bridge. I zoomed along the Brooklyn-Queens Expressway and reached the scene of Daniel's crash before the ambulances did. A cop car drove ahead of me. We weaved through the frozen traffic to the spot where the semitrailer stretched across the bridge. My tacos lay in the Styrofoam container beside me. Cold.

That day, I didn't get to eat my lunch, but I did get to do something more rewarding.

I jumped out of my truck and saw Daniel flat on his back on the road. Three firefighters knelt beside him with bare heads, their jackets off. They had smashed the windshield of the cab to pull him out. One firefighter, the heels of his palms on Daniel's chest, bobbed with the mechanical motion of CPR. A fire captain stood over them, timing the chest-compression cycles. Two minutes per rescuer. Lights flickered all around—red, yellow, white. An accident like Daniel's draws fire engines, fire trucks with ladders, ambulances, police cars. Highway police in knee-high boots held back the traffic. Firefighters steered a tow truck with a winch into place to right the semi.

I knelt beside Daniel. When I arrive at an emergency, I am the ranking medical officer, so I take charge of the medical situation.

"Lou, we pulled him out a few minutes ago," one of the firefighters said.

"He's not breathing," another one said.

"Keep up the compressions," I said. We needed a bag-valve mask so we could breathe for the patient. "Could you grab the BVM and the AED from the truck?" I asked one of the other firefighters.

Daniel was a burly guy, late forties. He wore a red flannel shirt. His baseball cap lay beside him on the asphalt. I cut open Daniel's shirt and undershirt with my Leatherman Raptors—shears that can cut through anything. In my truck, I had a basic automated external defibrillator, the kind you see in movie theaters and offices. The AED reads the rhythm for you and tells you if and when to shock the patient. Ambulance crews have a more sophisticated device that charts the heart rhythm with more specificity, but the ambulance hadn't arrived yet. So I made do with the machine on my truck.

The firefighter brought me the BVM and the AED; I stuck the pads on Daniel's chest, one under the right collarbone and the other on the lower left ribs. I turned on the machine. Told the firefighters to stop pumping.

Beeeep. "Analyzing," said a mechanical voice. Then: "Shock advised. Stand clear of the patient."

"Clear, clear," I said. "Everyone clear!"

The firefighters sat back on their heels. I pushed the button on the AED to deliver the shock. Daniel's body twitched as the machine zapped his heart. He was riding the lightning.

"Resume CPR," I said. More pumping. Two minutes. I held my fingertips to Daniel's neck. No pulse.

I reset the AED. Same cycle: Analyzing. Shock advised. Everyone clear. Shock delivered. Resume CPR.

After two more minutes, I held my fingers to Daniel's neck again.

"We got a pulse!" I said. There it was—a faint beat. The blood starting to flow through Daniel's vessels. And through my own body, a stab of adrenaline.

The firefighters looked up. "No shit. Really?" one said.

"Yep!"

The ambulance arrived; it had finally nudged its way through the logjam. We loaded Daniel onto a stretcher. He still wasn't breathing, so the paramedic crew intubated him. They ran a twelve-lead. It indicated a STEMI—an ST-segment elevation myocardial infarction, the most serious type of heart attack. Even more serious than the attack Joe had suffered. It meant that one or more of the arteries supplying blood to Daniel's heart were completely blocked. Part of his heart was getting no oxygen, and the muscle was dying.

"I'll send a note up to Staten Island North," I said. There was no traffic on the road heading to Staten Island. "He needs to go directly to the cath lab."

In the cardiac catheterization laboratory, they would perform an angiogram, pushing dye through the vessels in Daniel's heart to map the blood flow. They'd probably clear the artery using a little balloon threaded on a wire, then insert a stent to keep the artery open.

The ambulance pulled away. I turned to the firefighters who had been working on Daniel. "Great job, guys," I said. I shook their hands, then grabbed my defibrillator.

"You think he'll make it, Lou?" one of the firefighters asked. He sounded doubtful. But Daniel was fairly young. The pulse I'd felt on him was decent. The firefighters had reached him quickly.

"Yup," I said. "I think he will."

As I packed my gear into the truck, I smiled. Since Joe died, I'd had no energy at work. I wasn't buffing calls. I wasn't eager to be on the road. For the first time, I preferred to sit the desk at the station or watch the geese on the waterfront. But now I was elated. A guy in a flannel shirt would get to spend Christmas with his kids. He might live to be eighty. I felt like I was floating.

It was late afternoon and freezing cold, nothing like what I'd soon be experiencing Down Under, I told myself. The sky over Manhattan and New Jersey was orange and pink; the water below was dark. Cars crawled toward Brooklyn on the other side of the bridge. They slowed to look at the stranded semi. I'd have to drive to Staten Island and come back with the rubberneckers. Daniel was probably on his way into surgery. While they were fixing his heart, I'd be sitting in the traffic, staring at his trailer.

JANUARY 2020

I spent the first day of 2020 with Angie on Bondi Beach in Sydney, trying to get out of the New York state of mind.

We'd been in Australia for three days. My spirits had lifted the moment we got on the plane. Australia was the last continent on my list and on Angie's, so when we landed at Sydney Airport, we took a photo of our feet.

We'd timed our trip so we could be among the first people in the world to ring in the new decade. On New Year's Eve, we drank Bombay Sapphire gin and tonics from a can and watched the fireworks over Sydney Harbor. A security guard pointed us to a good viewing spot below the bridge there. It was fantastic. The fireworks burst over the opera house just like I'd seen on television.

On New Year's Day, we hit the beach. Bondi is a huge stretch of sand between two rocky headlands, a dramatic setting that sure beats the Rockaways. The ocean was full of people surfing and swimming; it seemed like half of Sydney was there. But we went in only up to our waists. I had expected the water to be calm, like the Caribbean. But the sea was cold and very fierce. I wouldn't swim in it even at my best, and now I had a weak arm to worry about.

A road ran along the back of the beach, and late in the afternoon, I spotted an ambulance parked there. Red and white checkers with a neon-yellow stripe. Tip-top condition.

Angie and I wandered over and introduced ourselves.

The paramedics were both male, one in his early fifties, the other in his thirties. They were lean and tan, like they'd just stepped off the set of *Baywatch*. The scene—buff medics, spiffy ambulance—was such a contrast to Brooklyn that it made me smile.

I asked what kind of calls they got.

"Intoxes, mostly," the younger medic said. "People who get legless on the beach." Drunk, in other words.

"Drownings," the older guy said.

"Any shootings?" I asked.

"Almost never," said the older guy. His last shooting had been a few years earlier. Mob-related incident. Red-light district. Shootings were rare, and this one was serious enough to make the papers, he said.

"That's how far back you have to go?" I asked. I was amazed. There are shootings pretty much every day in New York City. But it made sense. Australia has much stricter gun-control laws that we do.

Sometimes I feel foolish when I talk to emergency medical responders in other rich countries; I think they must feel sorry for us in New York. They have so much training, they're properly paid, and they have socialized medicine and sensible public safety laws. I remember meeting a group of medics in Helsinki who told me they earned forty-eight euros an hour. That works out to around twice what some of our paramedics make. It's about enough to buy a beer in Helsinki, but still.

The Australians said they had spent time in New York during their training. It turned out that New South Wales Ambulance sends trainees to cities like New York to get some action. These medics had ridden along on FDNY ambulances in Manhattan and Queens.

"New York was a hundred times busier than here," the older medic said. "I had no idea it would be so crazy!"

Angie and I laughed. At the time, we had no clue that EMS in New York was about to get busier and crazier than it had ever been.

We wished the guys a happy New Year and headed back to the sand. After all that followed—the chaos and sickness and death—I thought about those Australian paramedics. I wondered how things had gone for them. Better than they'd gone for us in New York, for sure. I imagine that they're still there, parked at the back of the beach, watching the surfers.

From Sydney, we flew to the outback in central Australia. There were wildfires raging in the southeast of the country, and our plane bounced up and down in the air because of all the heat rising from the flames.

We met up with a group in Uluru-Kata Tjuta National Park, home to Uluru, also known as Ayers Rock—a gigantic sandstone formation in the middle of a desert.

Our group was mostly Europeans in their twenties. We camped for five days. Slept on mattresses under the stars; built campfires; watched the sun come up. Uluru is famous for the way that it appears to change color as the light shifts through the day. The Aboriginal Australians believe the rock was created by spirits. That it's a living thing. That it talks to them.

Their myths are appealing. Living close to the earth, like the Aboriginals do, makes sense to me. It reminds me that I am part of a natural order and that nature can get along just fine without me.

As I walked around Uluru, I felt good about the fact that we had pulled off our trip. Made it to an amazing place that not many people got to see. Being in a wonderful natural environment replenished me. I couldn't control my job or the fact that the woman I was in love with was pulling away. But I still had this—sleeping under a huge sky and hiking in this landscape. The Buddha would tell me that I could find this replenishment anywhere; that there was no need for me to travel and that I could find peace inside me if I did the work. But sorry, Buddha—until I attain nirvana, I'm going to keep traveling.

On one of our last days in the outback, we went on a hike. We picked our way through a gully between huge boulders. Below us was a wide plain full of desert poplars, and beyond the plain we could see huge sandstone hills. Our guide, Ben, had explained that for the local people, the land was the source of everything they needed.

"What does it mean to you to be a Buddhist?" Ben asked. He was a young guy, very rugged, very thoughtful. Everything about him was coated in a thin layer of red dust—his hairline, the hem of his pants.

"Dude, this is Buddhism right here," I said. "Look around us. Everything is connected. Everything is in harmony. To me, Buddhism is just about being part of the natural world."

When we left the outback, we went to Melbourne. Melbourne was cosmopolitan, full of street art and hipsters and bars that made cocktails with elderflower liqueur. But smoke from the wildfires lay over the city. Some people wore masks to prevent smoke inhalation. One morning, the sky was so dark that I told Angie we should dress for rain.

From Melbourne, we flew to Auckland in New Zealand and drove north. We watched seals diving into the South Pacific and we walked through lavender fields, rows and rows of dark purple flowers that seemed to go on forever. I was stunned by the country's natural beauty. It was so lush, especially after the moonscape of the Australian outback. I thought about adding New Zealand to the tattoo on my left forearm that celebrates my travels, a globe surrounded by visa stamps from countries that I've visited. Mongolia, Iceland, Thailand, Egypt, Japan, Ecuador—those are the countries that have most impressed me. For its beauty, New Zealand tops them all.

We drove up the coast to Whangaruru, a community about three hours north of Auckland. Angie and I sat on the sand in a bay surrounded by green hills and fields that looked like velvet.

I looked out to sea. The water was bluish green. I wondered if my dad had ever crossed this expanse in his travels. He had sailed from Tokyo to Chile on one run, I knew, so he wouldn't have been far off.

My dad had a girlfriend in Japan. My mom found out about her because she wrote him letters. Very loving. In one of them, the girlfriend thanked my dad for helping to pay for her studies. That stung me more than the affair itself, since when I was looking at colleges, Dad steered me toward the places that were inexpensive. Even Hunter College, which is a state school, he considered too pricey. And yet he had money to pay for his girlfriend's studies. I didn't resent the girlfriend; I resented Dad for spending money on horses, on women, on things that were only for himself.

Still, I loved to tell Dad about my travels. He was interested in where I'd been, what I'd seen. Whenever I returned from a trip, my first phone call was to Dad.

I suppose that, in a way, I was Dad's favorite. We were both curious about the world. And when I was a kid, he liked that I studied and read and loved movies. He bought me speed-reading classes. Lent me books.

There was an element of complicity too. I kept Dad's secrets. The woman with the phantom ceiling fan. Other women. Even the time that he won $11,000 on a trifecta at Aqueduct.

I was eleven or twelve, and Dad had taken me to the races. He came back from the window with an enormous wad of cash. He slid out a hundred-dollar bill and handed it to me. "Don't tell your mom," he said. "She doesn't need to know how much we made."

When I got the medical job at Aqueduct in 2007, Dad told me, "Don't play the horses, Anthony. Don't gamble." He confided many things to me, but only he knew how much money he'd lost.

Dad and Yvonne didn't get along so well, I remember. Not by the time she was grown up, anyway. By then, Yvonne usually took Mom's side. Especially when it came to women. When I was ten years old, Dad had an affair with a woman named Ines who lived nearby. Ines was very nice to me. Always asked me questions. One day, Mom and Yvonne drove to Ines's house and waited for her to show up. When Ines pulled up in her car, Mom pounced and smashed her windshield with a baseball bat. They'd taken me with them. I watched everything from the back seat.

And with Richie, Dad simply lost patience. He never visited Richie in jail. I think he was ashamed. Dad didn't seem to mind when people cheated, but he wanted nothing to do with them when they got caught.

Morality was not the Almojeras' strong suit. My parents punished my siblings for bad behavior but behaved badly themselves. When Richie and Yvonne were young, Mom and Dad gave them the belt for lying; they made them kneel in rice if they filched things around the house. But when Richie, as an adult, stole a boxful of Nintendos, Dad happily kept one. Mom peeled stickers from items in the grocery store and replaced them with stickers for items that were cheaper; she stole cigarettes from the supermarket. It wasn't because she couldn't afford the things she wanted. We had money. But she got satisfaction from pulling a fast one on people.

My parents were less rigid with me than they were with my siblings. They'd slowed down by the time I came along. And they were usually too busy playing bingo or fighting to notice what I was up to. Not that I was up to anything much. I didn't take drugs and I worked for money rather than stealing it. The downside to this was that I often felt invisible. You didn't get a lot of attention in my family if you weren't fleecing Mom and Dad or shooting up drugs.

Richie monopolized Mom's attention even after he died. Grief drove her into the ground. She retreated into her relationship with Wilma, which lasted a few more years, on and off.

Eventually, Mom wound up under the same roof as Dad again. Dad moved to Philadelphia, and when his liver failed in 2002, Mom kicked out his crackhead girlfriend and moved in with him. She'd lost the two houses on Thirteenth Street because she'd stopped paying taxes. Then she'd moved upstate to some bungalows she owned there. She lost those too in the end.

Mom and Dad slept on separate floors of the house, just like old times. Mom saw Dad through his liver transplant. Then, in early 2005, she fell sick herself. She had a stroke, and her stint in the hospital revealed a string of maladies: High blood pressure. Diabetes. High cholesterol. The product of a life of high stress, poor diet, and almost no medical checkups. The doctors detected signs of prior transient ischemic attacks—mini-strokes where the blood supply to a part of the brain is briefly interrupted. And they said Mom needed triple bypass surgery.

Yvonne was living in Philly at that time. She'd built a family of her own with Joe, the guy she'd dumped Eddie, her first husband, for. They'd moved from city to city and from one failed business venture to the next. But they had three nice kids together, and Joe was a good stepdad to little Eddie. I would visit them now and then.

After Mom's bypass surgery, Yvonne and I decided to put her in a nursing home. She was only sixty-two, but she was showing signs of dementia, and she needed twenty-four-hour care. By the time she died, in 2013, she didn't recognize me.

In Whangaruru, as I stared at the sea, I thought about how my parents had brought me into the world and then expected me to muddle through with minimal guidance. "We didn't have to worry about you," Mom said a few years before she died. And now Mom, Dad, and Richie were gone. Yvonne was too, for all practical purposes—she and I hadn't spoken for a few years because we fell out over the way she handled money. And my parents had left me with nothing except an unpaid bill for Richie's funeral.

What was keeping me in New York? I thought. A job that was squeezing me dry? The promise of retirement pay? A rented apartment?

Friends, yes. But they could come and visit.

"Angie, we should come and live here," I said. "I'm serious."

We could go home for a few months to square things away, then head back to New Zealand. Angie was seeing a guy, Jonathan, in New York. Car salesman. Very easygoing. I knew this would make leaving complicated for her. But I figured that if I came up with a solid plan, I could convince her.

"We don't even have to be paramedics," I said. "We could open a pizzeria." That's my dream. A quiet life in a place of natural beauty running a bed-and-breakfast or a small restaurant. Somewhere I could be in charge of my own work schedule. Maybe meet a local woman. You never know.

If you retire from FDNY EMS after twenty-five years on the job, you receive half-pay for the rest of your life. That's enough to live on very comfortably in many of the places I've visited. In January of 2020, I was nine years away from this goal. But after seeing what had happened to Joe, I was starting to think about quitting the service sooner, about not waiting for that pot of gold at the end of the quarter-century rainbow.

Even as we sat on the beach talking about leaving New York, I knew we probably wouldn't do it. But I resolved to balance my life better in 2020. I'd exercise. Sleep properly. Get my arm fixed. Take better care of myself, even if that meant worrying about other people a bit less.

Unfortunately, the world had other ideas.

I'm a news junkie. I get the *Financial Times* delivered to my apartment and I leave it at work. Even when I travel, I listen to the BBC and Al Jazeera and read the *Economist*.

While we were in Australia, I started to see reports about an outbreak of a new coronavirus in Wuhan, China. Wuhan is bigger than New York City, but I'd never heard of it before January 2020. The virus was linked to a market that sold live animals. Dozens of people had been infected, but a health commission in Wuhan said there was no evidence that the virus could be spread by humans. Then a man from Wuhan died from the virus. He was sixty-one. He had underlying health conditions—a liver problem. He had often gone to the market to buy food.

While we were in New Zealand, a friend texted me about the outbreak. She was concerned that Angie and I would get caught in it. By that point, the Chinese government had locked down Wuhan and several other cities in the province of Hubei. There were hundreds of infections around the world. More than a dozen people had died. But they all seemed to be people who had been to Wuhan.

Don't worry! I texted back. China isn't near New Zealand!

She should look at a map, I thought.

In retrospect, there were omens: The wildfires. The smoke.

Then, as we waited in Auckland Airport to board our flight home, the screen of my phone lit up. Kobe Bryant had been killed in a helicopter crash with his daughter Gigi. She was thirteen years old. I couldn't believe it. Nobody could believe it.

"Angie," I said. "Kobe's dead.

"Man, this is some fucked-up start to the year."

A couple of days after we returned from New Zealand, I stood with my winter suntan at the bottom of a flight of stairs leading to the R train in Bay Ridge. I hopped from one foot to the other to stay warm. It was close to the end of January. The weather was mild by the standards of a New York winter, but to me, coming from the height of summer in New Zealand, New York felt frigid. And dark.

To add to the joy of my return to work, I was in a battle with Maribel. Maribel was one of the regulars. I'd known her for a few years. She was in her fifties. We'd picked her up drunk; we'd picked her up high. There were EMTs at my station who couldn't stand her. And I got it. She could be nasty.

We stood in a circle: me, Maribel, a cop, and a pair of pissed-off EMTs from Lutheran Hospital. I wasn't exactly on cloud nine either. The return to work had been jarring. I tried to take long vacations, European-style, so I could disengage. And I did. But the whiplash when I came home was rough. One day, I was in a coastal paradise in New Zealand; the next, I was at a Brooklyn subway stop with an irate addict. From the sublime to the R train.

Maribel shot the EMTs a sulky look. "They won't let me take my cart," she said. Maribel's cart was a constant source of tension with ambulance crews. It was stuffed with things that people had thrown away: An umbrella with a red handle and no fabric. Poland Spring bottles. Paper. Sheets of coupons. A plastic bag filled with clothes. One of the wheels was loose, and the cart tilted awkwardly. But where Maribel went, the cart went. It was a hoarder's den on wheels.

"Everything I need is in there," Maribel added. She had on a red headscarf and the long black overcoat she always wore. Garbage bags poked from the cuffs of her pants. She wore them wrapped around her legs, like plastic bloomers. I wasn't sure what their purpose was, but Maribel was adamant about keeping them. I heard that an ER nurse once tried to cut them off so she could dress a wound on Maribel's leg, and Maribel went berserk.

Maribel said she was born in the Bronx, but she seemed to live on the R train. She spent her days riding a loop between Thirty-Sixth Street and Fifty-Ninth Street. She would take a Manhattan-bound train from Fifty-Ninth Street and sit in one of the seats at the end of the subway car. She would get out at Thirty-Sixth Street and hang out on the platform. Then she'd take another subway back to Fifty-Ninth and start over.

But on this day, Maribel had been shouting at herself and at passengers near the subway entrance. One of the passengers alerted the transit police. A transit cop called EMS. Dispatch sent a crew from Lutheran Hospital, and they got into an argument about her cart.

"They always give me a hard time," Maribel rasped. She reeked of alcohol and urine. She asked the male EMT if he wanted oral sex in exchange for twenty bucks. He didn't respond. That was the kind of conversation you got from Maribel.

"It's okay, Maribel," I said. "We're going to take your cart with us."

That was what Joe Cengiz would have done. Joe never fought with an EDP. He knew there was no point. "Anthony," he'd say, "if they're not making any sense, what're ya gonna do? How you gonna argue with them?" To this day, if I have an EDP in an ambulance and that person tells me that people are following us, I play along. "Oh, yeah," I say. "I see them. But don't worry. You're safe here."

Dealing with EDPs is a valuable skill, and there are EMTs and paramedics who are true EDP whisperers. We have one at Station

40. He's fairly private. Reserved. But with an EDP, he's down on his haunches, speaking quietly, asking what's going on, and the next thing you know, the person is smiling, getting up, following him to the ambulance like a lamb. He doesn't judge the patient. He's not afraid or disgusted. He'd make a good Buddhist.

I grabbed Maribel's cart and pushed it toward one of the EMTs. "You take this," I said. Maribel's cart was heavy. I wasn't going to haul it. Not with my injury.

We headed toward the stairs. I figured that once the cart was moving, Maribel would follow. And she did.

Now the EMTs were giving *me* dirty looks. I couldn't blame them. The cart was probably teeming with germs. It might have had rotten food or soiled clothing in it. I wouldn't have wanted to put the cart in my truck either. But Maribel's insistence also made sense to me. She had no money, no home. She appeared to have no friends. Her cart and its collection of strange refuse was all she had.

Once the patient is in the ambulance, I normally peel off and let Dispatch know that I'm available. But this time, I followed the ambulance transporting Maribel to Lutheran. In the ambulance bay, I hopped out and reached for Maribel's cart. Maribel had her fingers around the handle like tentacles. She wouldn't let go. "I want to take it," she said.

"Maribel, we can't do that," I responded. "We have to leave it outside. Look," I said, pointing to a nook next to the emergency department where I would stash the cart. "When you come out, it'll be right there. I promise."

I walked ahead of Maribel to the emergency department's doors so she never lost sight of the cart. Then I stashed it in the nook.

As Maribel disappeared into the ED, I thought about how the system pushed her in circles: The MTA passed her on to the cops. The cops passed her on to EMS. EMS passed her on to the hospital. The hospital would send her back to the street. Subway, ambulance, emergency department, subway. A pointless loop, like the ones she made on the R train.

For some of the regulars, the loop was everything. Thomas, for instance. Thomas was another of our regulars, not a beloved one. He was a homeless guy in his mid-thirties who was emotionally disturbed, and he was bowlegged and very heavy, maybe three hundred pounds, so walking was extremely difficult for him.

Thomas hospital-hopped. He went from one emergency department to the next. He called 911 from his cell phone and said he was sick or that his legs were hurting him. We'd pick him up and take him to the ED. They knew him. Emergency departments keep a list of regulars with all their personal information; we don't even have to give them the patient-care report. The hospital staff was obliged to evaluate Thomas and stabilize him. But they were not obliged to treat him if he didn't have a medical emergency. So the staff gave Thomas a once-over and discharged him. He struggled down the street on his crooked legs and called another ambulance.

Thomas was an expert. He knew the rules. He knew that we wouldn't transport patients directly from one hospital to another. We would do that only if the hospital was on diversion—meaning it couldn't accept any more patients—or if the patient needed specialized treatment that the hospital couldn't provide. If you called us and you were on hospital premises or within a one-block radius of them, either we wouldn't pick you up or we'd drive you right back to the hospital. So Thomas would drag himself just far enough from the hospital and then call 911 again.

Not everyone is this savvy. We get plenty of perfectly sane patients who walk into the emergency department, get tired of waiting for treatment, walk out, and call 911 from the street outside the hospital. They believe that if we pick them up and bring them back to the same hospital, they will be treated more quickly. Same thing happens with emergency department patients who don't like the treatment they're receiving. They call 911 from one hospital in the hope that we'll transfer them elsewhere. No dice. Often, those people shouldn't be in an emergency department in the first place. They're using it as a primary care center, maybe because they have no insurance or because they don't understand how the system works. They jam up the ED and jam up our ambulance system. It's a huge waste of public resources, and it doesn't get anyone anywhere. It's its own kind of loop in a way.

The regulars we treated at Station 40 were scattered all over Brooklyn South, mostly on well-trafficked avenues and subway lines. I guess they knew that was where they could get food or alcohol or shelter. There was Sally, who wandered around Bay Ridge. Her body was mangled. She'd been hit by cars multiple times. The EMTs reckoned that she stepped out in front of vehicles on purpose for the insurance money. There was Yevgeny. He used to work as an engineer. Very intellectual. He'd written books on aerospace engineering. Now he was a drunk who muttered incomprehensibly.

Then there was Classic Tile. Classic Tile hung out in Bensonhurst, not far from where Joe lived. He was short, Latino, bad-tempered, and an alcoholic. Classic Tile wore a gray sweatshirt from the nearby tile store of the same name where he said he'd once worked. Classic Tile also claimed that he'd worked on the construction of the Twin Towers. It was very possible he did, but he didn't work on anything anymore.

Some days, Classic Tile was borderline comatose. Some days, he was mad. Often, we'd get calls from the MTA because was pissing on the wall of the subway station. He would take half-assed swings at the paramedics and EMTs who picked him up. He once flagged down Kenny's ambulance and then cursed blindly at him when he stopped. Kenny was one of the most good-natured EMTs you'd ever meet. He did not like Classic Tile.

Classic Tile had a raspy voice and three sentences in his repertoire. He flexed his arm, spat out a line, and slapped his biceps:

"I worked for Classic Tile. Twenty-five years." *Slap, slap.*

"I built the World Trade Center." *Slap.*

"I'm not a criminal." *Slap, slap.*

He was like a toy with a string that you could pull to make him talk.

Angie's favorite frequent flier was Dora. Dora was elderly, very petite. She lived in an assisted-living facility in Coney Island. Angie didn't work Coney Island, but she and Jimmy Mac were called to help Dora when there were no other ambulances in the area, which was fairly often.

Dora said she'd been a burlesque dancer when she was young. She wore very flamboyant clothes and colored pearls around her neck. Her makeup was outrageous. It looked like she applied it with a paint roller—lipstick all around her mouth, big blobs of rouge.

Dora called an ambulance every week. She was asthmatic and she had chronic obstructive pulmonary disease, COPD. It's actually a group of diseases, including emphysema, that cause your airways to become blocked. She always said she was having difficulty breathing. In reality, she was pissed at the staff at the living facility, and she wanted a change of scene. She'd ask the staff to fluff her pillows and they'd say no, so she'd call an ambulance. She figured that in the hospital, they'd fluff her pillows for her. She'd tell Angie all this. She was a pain in the ass. But she was a very sweet woman. Angie loved her.

When Angie and Jimmy showed up, Dora was usually out front waiting. She hopped right into the back. Angie assessed her, took her vitals. Dora was rarely sick. She overused her inhaler, which made her heart rate go up. The active ingredient in an inhaler, albuterol, works by relaxing the muscle in the airways. It allows more air to flow through. But it also stimulates the heart and makes it beat faster. This feels odd to the patient but it doesn't require treatment.

Sometimes Dora lay down on the stretcher and talked to Angie. Sometimes she danced in the back of the ambulance. Sometimes Angie fixed her makeup. "Look up, Dora," Angie would say. And she'd take surgical gauze and tidy up Dora's smudged eyeshadow or rouge.

One time, Dora said she'd lost her lipstick. Angie took her lip gloss out of her bag, cleaned the applicator with a disinfectant wipe, and handed the gloss to Dora.

"Keep it," she said.

It was tempting to get pissed at the regulars. They took up a lot of time. EMTs and medics are trained to restart people's hearts and treat gunshot wounds and save asthmatics from suffocating. But they spend much of their day wrangling people like Thomas and Maribel and Classic Tile.

Patients like these can be violent. They can be abusive. I've been punched in the face. I've been cursed at in a dozen languages. I've been peed on. The danger of working on an ambulance made headlines in March 2017 when Yadira Arroyo, an EMT with five children, was run over and killed by a mentally ill man who stole her ambulance. EMS workers' families aren't guaranteed line-of-duty death benefits, and Yadira's young family could have been ruined. The unions fought hard and helped push through a local law that stipulates three years' pay for a line-of-duty death. We needed the protection; after Yadira died, attacks on emergency medical workers continued to rise. There were a lot of unstable people in New York.

And while people like Maribel were a pain, she had a right to be pissed. Whatever safety net our society provided had failed to catch her. The closest Maribel came to any kind of care was getting a ride in the back of an ambulance with an EMT whose eyes watered from her stench and being given a sandwich when she was in the emergency department. Nobody talked to her. Nobody tried to peel off the layers of trauma and figure out what was going on. That would have taken people who were highly trained and extremely patient. And the city did not provide enough of those people.

Since I had joined the FDNY in 2004, the number of people sleeping on New York City's streets had grown and grown. Homelessness in 2020 was as bad as it was during the Great Depression. There wasn't enough affordable housing. There wasn't enough supportive housing, places where residents had access to social workers and mental health workers. Most of the homeless in New York were in shelters, but the number of people on the street had also grown. They often had issues like mental illness or addiction, which made them more likely to suffer physical illnesses—diabetes, hypertension. They were in and out of our ambulances all the time.

People like that shouldn't be judged. I'd like to say that Buddhism helped me realize this. Maybe it did. But growing up around my family also helped. I saw a bit of Almojera in many of the frequent fliers.

Take Patricia, the mother who lived in a mansion in Borough Park and called 911 for imagined maladies multiple times a week. She was a hypochondriac. I could identify with that. I spent much of my child-hood convinced that I was going to get AIDS. I didn't really know what AIDS was, but I knew that it happened to people like Donna, Cousin Victor, Aunt Barbara. My mom had taken me to the hospital to see Donna when she was sick. Donna was addicted to heroin. She was shrunken and thin, and her face was covered in lesions. We wore blue gowns and face shields to protect her from infection.

If AIDS could happen to her, I thought, couldn't it happen to me?

Later, when I started paying for sex, the possibility that I had gotten AIDS became logical to me. It also became a question of karma. I'd visited prostitutes, so I had it coming.

I recognize now that I was using sex the way other people use drugs or alcohol: To hide. To escape. The grief from Richie's death led to rages and bouts of depression, and the desire for physical contact became overwhelming, so when I didn't have a girlfriend, I would pay. I saw prostitutes for years. Not frequently—I couldn't afford it. But when I felt my mood sliding, that was where I turned.

Sleeping with those women fed my ego, my sense of prowess. I was a good lover, they said. One woman came to me and said she was get-ting out of the game but that she wanted to see me one more time. She didn't even want money. I couldn't believe it. A freebie from a woman who did this for a living! I should have been ashamed, but I was thrilled.

I ended up in counseling for sex addiction and I stopped seeing prostitutes more than eight years ago. There are times when I'm still tempted. When I'm desperate for comfort. But I'm like a recovering alcoholic—I know that one time would be enough to start the whole vicious cycle rolling again.

Even after I stopped paying for sex, the fear of AIDS stalked me. In early 2012, I collapsed and spent three days in the hospital. The doctors couldn't figure out what was wrong with me. They did blood tests, took stool samples. They asked if I'd had an HIV test. I freaked out. I had a low-grade fever, nausea, and diarrhea. All symptoms that you could have at the onset of AIDS—or a dozen other maladies.

Mike Sullivan took me to a clinic in Chelsea. Mike was a paramedic by then. He and I had remained close since we'd met as EMTs in Harlem. We'd traveled together—gone to Jamaica, Alaska, Montana, Ireland. We spoke every week, hung out as often as we could.

Mike and I got tested. I was shaking.

Mike whispered, "I know AIDS. And you don't have it."

Mike was right. I tested negative. It turned out I had giardia, which I'd picked up in India.

I felt so stupid. Mike had seen AIDS up close. He had lost friends to the virus. He was a sexually active gay man. He'd had the guts to get a test just to keep me company, and I was a ball of snot and tears and terror. A selfish idiot. But Mike was patient and understanding. If he thought I was being hysterical that day, he never said so.

A day or two after the incident with Maribel, the woman I had been dating for the past few months dropped by my apartment.

I lived in a one-bedroom in Midwood, in South Brooklyn. It was residential, middle class, quiet. Detached houses with small, neat lawns out front. My apartment was at the top of a yellow house with a cherry tree in the yard. In 2009, I moved there from my first apartment, the studio in Borough Park that I rented when I first joined the FDNY after two years without a roof over my head.

My apartment wasn't fancy, but it had character: hardwood floors, sloped ceilings, blue and brown and ocher walls. (I painted.) It was spacious and tidy. I'd added more plants to go alongside the philodendron.

At the top of the stairs that lead into the apartment, I had framed photos of the Group Home. There were pictures of Angie, Kala, Mike. Mike was a good-looking guy. Tall and trim. There was a photo of me in New Orleans with Johana Clerge, who trained with me as an EMT at the FDNY academy. She was a lieutenant at another Brooklyn station. Extremely competent. In 2013, I invited Johana and a bunch of friends to New Orleans to scatter my father's ashes with me. Bought everybody flights. We turned it into a celebration. I spread half the ashes on the street in the French Quarter, where my dad was raised, and the other half I scattered on Lake Pontchartrain, which had burst over levees during Hurricane Katrina and flooded New Orleans in 2005. I went to the edge of Pontchartrain, where it lets out to the sea. Dad loved working on the ocean, so the spot felt fitting.

There was another picture with Wes—a friend I made in Montana who later became a medic—and his wife, Jessa, when we got together for their wedding in Hawaii. I was living in my car at the time. Marshall paid for my ticket. Wes thanked me in his speech because I was homeless but I'd still made it to Maui. I was touched and a little embarrassed. Wes and Jessa were still married, still glowing. The happiest couple I knew.

Most of my Group Home friends were marked by loss—an absent parent, a sibling who'd died. We swapped ACE (adverse childhood experiences) scores the way other friends talked about SATs or what they bench-pressed. Dre's dad bailed on him when he was a kid; so did Manny's. Mike, me, Angie, and our friend Pete Borriello, a goodhearted curmudgeon who was a lieutenant at Station 39, had all lost a brother when we were young. (Pete's brother died of non-Hodgkin's lymphoma at seventeen.)

Instead of becoming mean and bitter, they were the friendliest, kindest, most loyal people imaginable. They took their pain and channeled it into helping people. They tried not to repeat the mistakes of their parents. It wasn't smooth sailing. But they—we—muddled along. We got out the duct tape and the Krazy Glue and tried to stop the toys from falling apart.

The woman I'd been dating went straight into the kitchen. It was big enough to eat in—a distinction in New York—with a big Le Creuset cooking pot and fridge magnets from dozens of countries.

We were still "on a break," as she put it. We hung out, but less often than we used to.

I resisted the urge to make a move. I made her a drink. She asked about my trip. She looked very pretty.

We went into the living room. I hovered near the window. She sat on the IKEA chair.

"I always found that couch too soft," she said. She gave me a coy look. We'd had sex on the couch. A lot.

"I'm sorry," I said. "I don't remember that being a problem."

She laughed. "Best sex I have ever had," she said.

I felt my face catch fire. And then she got up and put her arms around my neck and kissed me.

FEBRUARY 2020

Tons of people came to watch the parade for Chinese New Year in Lower Manhattan. I walked along with a river of marchers snaking through Chinatown. The streets were lined with spectators squeezed behind police barriers waving Chinese and American flags.

It was February 9. Since I'd returned from vacation, there had been a lot of chatter about the coronavirus. Donald Trump had banned non-Americans who had traveled through China from entering the United States. Thousands of people were quarantined aboard a cruise ship, the *Diamond Princess,* in Yokohama Bay in Japan. Hundreds of people in China had died. A man who'd traveled from Wuhan to the Philippines was the first person to die of the virus outside China—or at least, the first person whose death was reported. A young Chinese doctor who'd tried to warn people about the outbreak in Wuhan had also died. Before the man's death, the Chinese authorities had made him retract his warning and say it was just a rumor.

It was clear we couldn't trust the Chinese government to be transparent about the virus. But banning people who had traveled to China was stupid, I thought. Very xenophobic. Our president was a fearmonger. The virus was a pretext for him to score points against China and stigmatize people of Chinese descent in the United States. That shit wasn't going to fly with me. I worked in a Chinese community and

I was fond of the people there. I wasn't about to avoid a Chinese celebration because of hype about a virus, so I joined the parade.

We walked with the Phoenix Society, an FDNY association for Asians and Asian-Americans. The society represented the department in the parade, and I'm a member. We were a pretty small group. People of Asian descent make up only 5 percent of the EMS workforce and 2 percent of the fire department as a whole. That's in a city that's about 14 percent Asian.

The fire department is the least diverse of the uniformed services in New York. If you leave out EMS, it's 99 percent male and 77 percent white. The EMS division, by contrast, is 72 percent male and 41 percent white. One of the things that the fire department did by taking over EMS was boost its department-wide diversity numbers. But they're still shameful. In 2014, the FDNY's hiring practices were found to be discriminatory, and the city council passed a law forcing the department to report on the demographics of its applicant pool. That way, the city could see whether minorities were applying to join the department and at which point they were being rejected.

Even with the extra scrutiny, the city still gets complaints about the racist and sexist culture at fire stations. In 2019 the department settled at least two discrimination cases, one brought by a male Muslim firefighter who was subjected to racist bullying and one brought by a male firefighter who alleged that other firefighters bullied him, vandalized his car, and used homophobic and racist slurs. The year before, there'd been an outcry after a firefighter allegedly called an African-American EMT a Black bitch—he'd managed to be racist and sexist in a single phrase.

At the parade, nobody seemed fearful of the coronavirus. There hadn't been any confirmed cases of the virus in the state. Very few people wore masks. The ground was red with confetti, and a long green dragon made of silk or paper bobbed above the marchers. A woman on a float held a sign that said STAY STRONG, CHINA.

Standing on a podium, Bill de Blasio said that the city was vigilant. That he stood with the people who were facing the virus in China.

Congresswoman Nydia Velázquez told the crowd that the city had confronted other virus outbreaks and that we'd successfully confront this one. She said she'd eaten in a Chinese restaurant the night before. "Chinatown is open for business," she said. "We are behind you, and we will remain strong."

I walked in the parade with my friend Terence Lau, the paramedic I'd traveled with to Hong Kong in November. His girlfriend, Vanessa, also came; so did Angie's roommate, Kala.

We started marching on Mott Street, went under the Manhattan Bridge, then up toward the Bowery. We held Roman candles that sprayed sparks above our heads. I shook hands with everybody.

It felt good. We were showing solidarity. We were showing that we weren't nervous.

Of course, if we'd known then what we know now, we'd have been very nervous indeed.

Like so many New Yorkers, I found it hard to believe that the city could end up like Wuhan. But I did know one thing. If the virus spread here, EMS would be the tip of the spear defending the community. And we weren't in good shape for battle.

About a week before the parade, I had said as much to the FDNY brass and a group of city council members when I testified at City Hall before the New York City Council Committee on Fire and Emergency Management. The committee members sat at a big horseshoe-shaped table in a hearing room with mint-colored walls and chandeliers. Four union bosses, including me, sat facing them.

The hearing was about attrition and low pay, issues that affect emergency medical services all over America. The World Health Organization says EMS is essential to integrated health care, yet city after city invests little in its emergency medical services. We're a young profession. We don't have the recognition—good or bad—that cops and firefighters have. We often feel invisible.

In New York, the issue was finally getting attention. Yadira Arroyo's death had people talking about the dangers of the job and about the poor benefits. In the fire department family, EMS workers were the poor cousins. A firefighter's base pay at the time started just shy of $44,000 per year and rose to $85,292 after five years; an EMT started at a base salary of $35,000 that rose to $50,604 after five years. A paramedic's base salary peaked at $65,226.

We'd been told by New York officials that our pay was different because our jobs were different. On the surface, that was true; firefighters fight fires, and emergency medical workers deal with medical emergencies.

But that wasn't the full story. Firefighters in many parts of the United States spend as much time on medical calls as they do on fighting fires. In 2018, for example, FDNY firefighters responded to about 600,000 incidents. Half of them were medical, and less than 10 percent were fires.

New York firefighters are highly skilled at preventing and extinguishing fires. But they're not especially skilled at responding to medical emergencies. At the time of the hearing, their training consisted of an eighty-hour first-responder course. FDNY EMTs, by contrast, received at least thirteen weeks of training. Paramedics went to school full-time for a year. If you crashed your car and found yourself surrounded by firefighters, EMTs, and paramedics, the responders with the least medical training would probably be the firefighters. And they were the ones earning the most money.

The FDNY argued that sending fire trucks to medical emergencies was the fastest way to reach patients. That was true. At that point, there were two hundred fifty fire stations and thirty-seven EMS stations. EMS couldn't cover the ground as quickly as firefighters could. And firefighters were less stretched than we were. Compared to the 600,000 incidents that FDNY firefighters clocked in 2018, EMS responded to 1.5 million.

But using fire trucks costs the taxpayer a lot of money. A study in 2018 estimated that each fire-engine run in New York City cost about four times as much as each ambulance run. Ambulances can charge patients' insurance for transporting them to the hospital. Fire engines don't transport patients, so they can't charge. Ambulances are the FDNY'S breadwinners.

Big cities like Los Angeles and Chicago have trained their fire-fighters to be EMTs and paramedics. Paramedic-firefighters in Seattle have to complete a year of emergency medical training and do fifty hours of medical education annually to keep their certification. I don't think this is the solution. To master the job of being either a firefighter or a paramedic takes years. You shouldn't try to do both. Firefighters don't want to run medical calls. And they shouldn't have to. What makes sense is increasing the size of EMS.

At the hearing, dozens of EMS workers stood at the back of the room. They held up signs that read EQUAL PAY FOR EMS. Over a hundred more crammed themselves into a bar across the street and asked the bartender to tune into the live broadcast of the hearing.

City council member Justin Brannan said that the FDNY's EMTs and paramedics were leaving for cities where they were treated better.

"We like to think that we're the greatest city in the world," he said, "but other cities are eating our lunch."

Committee members grilled Lillian Bonsignore, the FDNY's chief of EMS. Chief Bonsignore, an openly gay single mom, was the first female chief of EMS. She'd seemed like a breath of fresh air when she was put in charge of the force in May 2019. But she hadn't come through for us. She'd gotten caught up in the politics of the job.

Question: How many EMS workers left each year to join fire suppression, (the firefighting side of FDNY)?
Answer: Twenty-two percent every four years.
Question: What percentage of the EMS force has less than a year on the job?

Answer: Thirteen percent.

Question: Is thirty-five thousand dollars a livable wage in New
York City?

Answer: We don't have the ability to make that judgment.

That was a kick in the gut. There are studies that show that a working adult in New York City with no children needs about $45,000 a year to live. The chief had a chance to stick up for her coworkers, but she chose not to.

I spoke on behalf of my union, Local 3621. I wore a dark blue suit, Manchester United cuff links, and a Brooks Brothers tie with kangaroos on it. I make sure I look sharp when I represent the union. (My father never dressed well; he always wore cheap knockoffs and shoes that fastened with Velcro. Not me.)

Chief Bonsignore's remarks had pissed me off. I pointed out that the city shoots itself in the foot by paying EMS workers so little that they leave to become firefighters or join other uniformed services. Over the past four years, I said, 68 percent of EMS personnel had quit or left to become firefighters or cops or sanitation workers. As a result, the average New York City EMS employee had about four years on the job.

"The citizens of NYC and all those who visit deserve a fully invested, compensated, and independent EMS workforce," I said.

I could hear my voice getting tight. I get emotional about the raw deal that EMS workers get. I love EMS and I know how good it could be if we held on to people. But fire suppression gives priority to FDNY EMS workers if they want to join. The policy bleeds the service of EMTs and paramedics. They spend a few years in EMS and then become firefighters. It's such a waste of medical training. A paramedic in a firefighter's uniform is no longer considered a paramedic. They're not allowed to provide advanced life support. They have all that knowledge, and they can't use it.

I understand why people switch to fire suppression. I nearly did. In 2007, I was accepted into the fire department's fire-suppression training

program. I quit the emergency medical service and enrolled in the academy on Randall's Island. I lasted three days.

A firefighter yelled at me as I walked to the academy. "What are you
doing on my sidewalk?" he shouted. "You walk in the street." Apparently,
only firefighters walk on the sidewalk. Cadets walk on the street.

"But there are cars in the street," I said. Ever the smart-ass. "Isn't it
dangerous to walk there?"

In the classroom, the drill instructors wanted us to sit in a specific
position: arm on the leg, elbow flush with the hip, hand cupping the
knee. It was awkward because the desks were very cramped and I'm
relatively tall. One of the drill instructors yelled at me to sit properly.
I asked him how old he was. He said he was twenty-six. I was thirty.
I was a qualified paramedic. I thought, *Fuck this shit*. I wasn't mad at
him. He was doing his job. Instructors try to weed out the applicants
whose hearts are not really in it. People like me. On the fourth day, I
pulled aside the instructor and asked if it was too late for them to give
my spot to a different EMS candidate.

The drill instructor said it wasn't too late. But he shook his head.
"You're making the biggest mistake of your life," he said.

"Maybe," I said. "But it's my life."

Firefighting wasn't for me. EMS is more freewheeling. We have
protocols and rules, and we follow them. But we want people who
can act independently. The fire-suppression side, by contrast, is very
hierarchical. It's like a fraternity. They haze the rookies. The department was sued in 2017 over an incident of sexual hazing. A rookie was
made to lie faceup on a workout bench while a naked firefighter held
his genitals near his face. I'm a good-natured person; if I'm new to a
station, I'll bring food the first day or I'll do the dishes. I'll follow the
rules of the house. But if you try and strap me down and put your balls
in my face, you'd better run. Very fast.

Even though I mainly talked about pay parity at the hearing, I made
a reference to the virus. I warned them: "It will be EMS on the front
line, treating and containing it."

EMS workers would fly blind into the fray, I said, because "we know our sacrifice will help protect and save the lives of the people in this great city."

My comments sound prescient now. But if I'm honest, I had no idea if the virus would hit us. Or what would happen if it did.

I had worked through other virus outbreaks, outbreaks that spooked people but never took root in the United States. Not long after I became an EMT, severe acute respiratory syndrome spread around the globe. The illness is caused by a coronavirus called SARS-associated coronavirus, or SARS-CoV. It's very deadly. It infected about eight thousand people and killed nearly eight hundred, according to the official count. But it barely grazed the United States.

Then there was the 2009 H1N1 pandemic—the swine flu. The swine flu killed thousands of people in the United States and sent places, like Mexico City, into lockdown. But it probably claimed no more lives than seasonal flu.

The scariest was the Ebola outbreak that began in 2014 and killed thousands of people in West Africa. There were very few cases in the United States, but the illness is so terrifying that the fire department performs an Ebola drill twice a year.

For these Ebola drills, we gather in a big training room at the EMS academy in Fort Totten in Queens and sit through a presentation on the disease and how to identify it. We go over the protocols that we should follow if we pick up a suspected case.

We practice suiting up with personal protective equipment. It's hard core. Ebola spreads through direct contact with the infected person's bodily fluids—vomit, saliva, blood, sweat. So protecting yourself from an Ebola patient means covering up from head to toe. We put on Tychem suits—hooded coveralls made from polyethylene-coated Tyvek. The coveralls have taped seams, a flap down the front to prevent anything from penetrating the zipper, and elasticized wrists to prevent exposure of the skin between your gloves and your forearms.

You pull on a pair of gloves and then slip your arms into the sleeves of the coverall. Then you pull on yellow rubber boots and an escape mask with filters on either side of the jaw. Finally, you pull on a second pair of gloves. Donning the suit properly takes about ten minutes. Once you're suited up, you feel like a piece of meat swaddled in six layers of Saran Wrap. It's incredibly hot. It traps your sweat.

There's a meticulous procedure for taking off the protective gear after you've treated a patient: Peel off the left sleeve of the gown, grab the left wrist of the gown and the wrist of the outer glove, and pull them off in one movement. Pull the right sleeve off by grabbing it from the inside of the gown; repeat the process of taking off the outer glove and sleeve together. Roll them up and put them in a biohazard bag. Next, remove shoe coverings by placing your gloved hands inside them and rolling them off. Put those in the biohazard bag. Remove the gloves and put on a fresh pair before you remove your mask. Remove the gloves and discard in the biohazard bag. Wash your hands and face.

Because of the drills at Randall's Island, I assumed there was an enormous storage facility somewhere in Queens that was full of the equipment that we would use during a pandemic. I had a vision of the massive warehouse in *Raiders of the Lost Ark,* the one where the wooden crates are piled high in stacks that go on forever. Looking back, though, I realize that those supplies were actually more like the Ark of the Covenant in that movie: a single box hidden in the endless stacks where nobody could find it.

Around the time of the hearing at City Hall, the fire department gave the new coronavirus its own call type: fever/cough. Two words that were as vague as our understanding of the virus was. They would echo through our lives for a long time to come.

An internal memo instructed dispatchers to add the words *fever/ cough* to the call type of a patient who might have the 2019 novel coronavirus: sick, fever/cough; arrest, fever/cough; diff breather,

fever/cough; and so on. That way, the EMTs and paramedics responding to the call would know that their patient was potentially infectious.

A fever/cough patient was described in the memo as someone who
had a fever *or* a cough *and* who had traveled to China or had had
contact with someone who'd been there. When the crew transported
the patient, they should use the fever/cough designation to alert the
hospital. Within weeks, it became clear that the China connection was
irrelevant, and the instructions were revised—any patient with a fever
or a cough was given the designation, no matter where that person
had traveled or who he or she had had contact with.

"Four-Two X-Ray," the paramedic might say. "Notification to Fifty-One.
Fifty-two-year-old male. Diff breather. Fever/cough. BP one forty over
eighty, pulse one hundred and fourteen, respirations twenty-four and
labored. ALS established. ETA to hospital Fifty-One approximately
eight minutes."

The same memo instructed every EMT and paramedic who transported a patient with suspected coronavirus to wear gloves, a gown,
goggles or a face shield, and an individually fitted N95 mask, then
throw everything away after each patient contact.

Every EMT and medic is supposed to have a supply of N95s that
fits him or her. The fire department tests the fit of the mask annually to make sure you know what size to wear. As part of this test, you
put on a mask and a hood. The person helping to fit the mask sprays
around your head with something that smells bitter and lemony. Not
in a nice way. If you can smell the spray, the mask doesn't fit properly.
They adjust it until you can't smell anything. If they can't fit the mask
on you properly—because of facial hair or some other reason—you are
supposed to wear a hood and respirator.

In the memo, the health department recommended that ambulances
be aired out for two hours after every fever/cough call.

Two hours. That seems laughable now.

Last, the memo instructed members to consult with the online medical control unit—telemetry—if they had a patient with a suspected

case of novel coronavirus. The EMTs or medics would call the doctor, and the doctor would direct them to a hospital with the capacity to isolate and test the patient.

The hospital that traditionally dealt with patients who required isolation was Bellevue. That's where New York's first Ebola patient was treated in 2014. He was a doctor, Craig Spencer, who had been treating Ebola patients in Guinea. Mike Sullivan, my Group Home friend, was one of the medics who transported the sick doctor to the hospital. At the time, Mike was working in a unit that specialized in incidents involving hazardous substances. Their ambulances are equipped with gear such as breathing apparatuses and Tychem suits. They have hoses and decontaminating solutions for cleaning off the ambulance and themselves after they transfer a patient. Mike and his colleagues put an oxygen mask on the patient and covered him with sheets to try to prevent him from spreading the virus. The fire department set up portable showers at Bellevue, and once the crew had transferred the patient, they were decontaminated, and the ambulance was taken out of service. When you have a single contagious patient, those are the lengths you can go to.

Other than the memo, there was little discussion at the fire department about what we should do to prepare. We weren't told to check on our stocks of masks. We weren't told to hold drills to make sure the EMTs and paramedics understood the protocols. There was nothing about getting additional supplies of personal protective equipment. Just one memo describing a meticulous protocol that we'd soon learn was a fantasy.

A few days after the Chinese New Year parade, Angie started feeling bad. She had a sore throat and a low-grade fever. But she kept working. Angie rarely gets sick, and when she does, she doesn't stay home. She believes that sick days are for going to the beach.

New York City EMS workers get twelve paid sick days per year. We've been fighting to get unlimited sick leave; that's what cops and firefighters and sanitation workers get. We treat people with illness and infection all day long. It's only reasonable that we should get the same sick leave as other uniformed services. But we don't. So unless Angie feels terrible or has something that might infect others, she keeps going to work.

One afternoon not long after Angie fell sick, she was coming down from the locker room on the second floor of the station and the station captain saw her. He told her she looked terrible and that she should go home.

There was no question of Angie being tested for coronavirus. Nobody in EMS was getting tested. When Angie got sick, there still hadn't been a confirmed case of coronavirus in New York State. The virus had only days before been given a name by the International Committee on Taxonomy of Viruses: severe acute respiratory syndrome coronavirus 2, or SARS-CoV-2. The World Health Organization had named the disease that the virus caused COVID-19, for "coronavirus disease 2019."

Angie went to CityMD, an urgent-care clinic. She has a physician, but in a city that's as densely populated as New York, it can take over a week to get an appointment. At CityMD, you can just walk in and be seen. Our insurance through FDNY covers treatment, but you have to pay fifty dollars out of pocket per visit.

By American standards, EMS workers get decent health-care coverage. The co-pays are not too high, though that fifty-dollar out-of-pocket charge is about two hours' pay for a lot of EMTs. There are so many city workers on the plan that plenty of doctors accept our insurance. But not all. And it's no substitute for universal health care, which is a dream I have that I doubt I'll ever see come true.

At CityMD, they swabbed Angie for strep throat. Negative. They tested her for mononucleosis. Negative. They gave her a Z-Pak—azithromycin, an antibiotic that's often used to treat strep and bacterial pneumonia. And they sent her home.

A medic from the station drove Angie back to her apartment. She fell asleep on the couch. Her fever rose to 100 degrees. Then 101. Then 104. She sweat through her hoodie. Her body ached. She showed Kala, her roommate, how to start an IV, and Kala hooked her up to a bag of fluid.

I texted Angie: Don't die of coronavirus! Then: I wonder if you've got this thing?

A few days later, Angie returned to work. She was fatigued and felt run down, but she didn't want to waste those beach days.

Later that week, I was at Lutheran Hospital and bumped into one of my teachers from paramedic school, Tony Thomas.

I was on what we call "bay watch." Not the kind that involves lifeguards with great bodies diving into the surf to save people. The chiefs like the lieutenants to check on crews in hospital ambulance bays—the zones where the ambulances park to transfer patients. If it's taking a long time to transfer patients, lieutenants talk to the ER staff to try and hurry things along. EMS is permanently short-staffed, so we can't afford to have ambulance crews twiddling their thumbs in the emergency bays. The chiefs also want us to make sure our crews aren't just killing time after they drop a patient. I'm less of an enforcer in that regard. The guideline is half an hour—pee, get something to drink in the cafeteria, and wipe down your ambulance, then hit the button on the screen to signal that you are clear for your next assignment.

I was talking to an ambulance crew when I heard someone call my name and turned to see Tony. He was a terrific instructor; I don't know if I'd have passed my paramedic course without him. I was squeezing in classes and rotations while working full-time as an EMT, and Tony would go over things with me after class.

"Tony! I thought you retired," I said.

This was a running joke between us. He had been on the job for thirty-five years. When I met him, he had a thick head of wavy hair. Now he had a shiny bald head and a gray mustache. Every time I saw him, he swore to me that he was about to retire. But here he was, finishing up the overnight tour at Lutheran. Seeing Tony made me think of Joe. It also reminded me that I didn't want to wind up bald and still grinding away.

"Almost there," Tony said. "Almost there."

"Almost where? You should be in the Philippines on a beach," I said. "Man, you need to stop!" Tony had a lovely wife from the Philippines. He talked about going there to live. But every year he worked, his retirement fund grew. So he kept working.

"I know," Tony said. "Almost there."

During the second half of February, the rumble of coronavirus became louder. On February 14, an elderly woman died of the virus in France—the first person to die of the novel coronavirus outside Asia. A day or two after that, the U.S. government sent cargo planes and doctors in hazmat suits to extract about four hundred American passengers from the *Diamond Princess*.

And then Italy locked down Lombardy, a region in the north of the country. Now there were more cases in Italy and Iran than in China. The virus was clearly hopping borders.

The lieutenants at Station 40 began putting members on alert. Our station was in the middle of one of the biggest Chinese communities in New York City. Sunset Park and Borough Park rival Lower Manhattan for the size of their Chinese population. If an infected traveler from China landed in New York, there was a decent chance he or she would head straight to our neighborhood.

We had roll call at the beginning of every eight-hour tour, a meeting where the lieutenant on duty updated the units about anything that was going on and went over housekeeping issues. The items were usually mundane: Hospital 51 is on diversion; watch out for the broken traffic light on the corner of Sixty-Fifth Street and Thirteenth Avenue; there's a new CME—continuing medical education—unit on the computer that you need to complete.

During one of the roll calls I led around this time, I raised the issue of coronavirus. Even then, it wasn't on the top of the agenda. We didn't want to be alarmist.

"Kenny, can you and your partner please make sure that you guys are hitting your eighty-nine? We're getting calls that you guys were ninety-seven for two hours."

An ambulance is supposed to return to its intersection—its eighty-nine—between calls. The code for being in the service area but away from the eighty-nine is ten-ninety-seven.

"Sure, Lou."

"Four-Two Adam, I need you guys to submit your time sheets. You guys are off tomorrow. End of the week. Get your time sheets in.

"Also, a heads-up: the new coronavirus. We don't know much about it. We don't really know what it looks like. But we do know that it originated in China and that we serve a Chinese community. I want you to look out for anything unusual. You know what PPE you need to protect yourselves from infection. Take a mask with you. Use it if you have any doubts. Use the fever/cough call type if you think you have a case. Any questions?"

"There's no way that I am going to catch the coronavirus."

That was from Arnold Chen, one of the EMTs. Very health-conscious. Ate well. Arms like pythons. Chen liked to joke about how many germs EMTs and paramedics were exposed to.

"I've had every disease in the book," he said.

Bones was also unruffled. A two-decade EMS veteran, he never got sick. He was convinced it was because he ate a lot of broccoli rabe. That was the Brooklyn Italian in him, I guess.

"I am immune to everything," Bones said.

We laughed. None of us knew just how much we were tempting fate.

As the days passed, the warnings became more ominous. On February 25, Benjamin Haynes, a spokesman for the Centers for Disease Control and Prevention, said that community spread was inevitable.

"It's not so much a question of if this will happen anymore but rather more a question of exactly when this will happen and how many people in this country will have severe illness," he said.

He talked about social-distancing measures like closing schools, working from home, canceling mass gatherings.

"I understand this whole situation may seem overwhelming and that disruption to everyday life may be severe," he said. "But these are things that people need to start thinking about now."

I didn't dismiss these warnings. I believed that the virus would hit New York. But I didn't think the city would come to a standstill. I remember telling people that.

Toward the end of February, I was working a shift at Aqueduct when an old man got sick. Aqueduct Racetrack is in Ozone Park in Queens. It's the only racetrack in New York City. I work there once a week as part of a team of medics who are on standby in case a jockey gets hurt or a spectator has a stroke.

Aqueduct is run-down and dingy. There's a group of people who come every day. They're crazy about the races, and they're mainly gambling addicts. After the live racing finishes for the day, the hardcore gamblers go into the building and watch races at other tracks around the country on a bank of televisions upstairs.

It was evening. The elderly man was sitting on the floor of the lobby, a security guard crouching next to him. The guard told me that the guy was ninety-six and that his name was Samuel.

"But I like to be called Sam," the old man said.

"Okay, Sam. Nice to meet you. How are you doing?"

Sam said he had chest pain. Upset stomach. I took his pulse and his blood pressure. Pressure was 124/80. Slightly above normal for a guy his age. He looked pretty fit to me. I figured he had indigestion. I told him we'd get him an ambulance so that he could go and get checked out, just in case. We called 911.

While we waited for the ambulance, I chatted with Sam. I love chatting to old people. They have so many stories. Sam had been coming to

Aqueduct for seventy-five years. He'd come home from World War II, he said, and started betting on horses.

Sam lived in Queens. He took the A train to the racetrack every day. He put a dime on any horse he liked.

"Sam, do you ever win big?" I asked.

"Sometimes I do," he said.

"What's the most you've ever won?"

He smiled. "Two dollars and seventy cents."

Sam was well turned out: Big flat cap. Trousers that were on the loose side. He still had some of his hair. I told him I thought he was very well dressed.

"I always try to look presentable," he said.

Sam said he didn't have any family. His wife had died twenty years ago, and they didn't have kids.

I walked Sam down to the ambulance. We put him on a stretcher and wheeled him into the bus.

"Anthony, am I going to be okay?" Sam asked.

"You're gonna be fine, Sam," I said. "You're in very good hands."

I nodded to the FDNY EMTs, an older guy and a young woman, who were settling him into the back of the ambulance.

"What do you think about this virus?" Sam said. "Do you think they'll close down the track?" He looked concerned. "If I can't come here, I don't know what I'll do every day."

"Don't worry, Sam," I said. "I'll see you here next week."

I guess I was in denial. I think a lot of people were. Even as late as the end of February, I didn't think the virus would be a huge deal. And while I waited to see what would happen, there were bargains to be had. Flights had become ridiculously cheap because people were afraid to travel. So less than a month after I returned from New Zealand, I started planning my next trip.

Looking back, I see how shortsighted I was—how shortsighted we all were. I was taking advantage of cheap flights and theater tickets instead of preparing for what was to come. We were like the coastal villagers who'd run onto the beach just before the tsunami hit Southeast Asia in December 2004. They'd watched the water recede from the beach and they'd seen all the fish stranded on the sand. They didn't know what to make of the low tide, didn't realize that it signaled disaster, so instead of running to safety, they'd gone onto the beach to gather up the free fish.

I spent one morning searching the internet for flights to Luanda, the Angolan capital. I was curious about Angola. What kind of place would it be after so many years of war? I also wanted to go to Namibia, to Angola's south. I wanted to see the huge sand dunes and the Himba, a nomadic people who live in northern Namibia. The Himba women cover their skin and hair in a paste made with red ocher. On the internet, I found a guide who said he could take us to see them.

I called Angie.

"We could get to Angola for six hundred and twenty. Round trip."

"You're shitting me," Angie said.

"Nope."

"Hang on. Remind me, where would we be flying to?"

"New York to Luanda. Cross the border into Namibia by land. Fly out of Windhoek."

"For six twenty? Are you serious?" Angie said.

"I am."

"I'm down!"

For people who weren't afraid of coronavirus, the end of February was the beginning of a brief bonanza. You could fly practically anywhere on the globe for next to nothing. I read about millennials heading to Barbados or Mexico for cheap holidays. I wasn't planning to go anywhere till the summer, but I wanted to lock in the cheap airfare.

Uncertainty about the virus was creating all kinds of opportunities. Stores that still had supplies of toilet paper and Lysol wipes had jacked up their prices. Property owners in upstate New York and Long Island raised their rates as affluent Manhattanites hunted for places to sit out the pandemic. (If New York was going to be shut down, they had no desire to be shut down with it. They figured—correctly—that they'd be better off in the country.) Everyone was looking for an angle.

And my angle was a $620 flight to Angola. I was so excited by the airfare that my hands shook.

I called Mike and told him how inexpensive the flights were. Mike always takes a little more convincing than Angie, who is game for pretty much anything. She and I started going on trips together in 2017. Our first journey was to Colombia. Angie hadn't traveled much beyond the Caribbean at that point. While Angie and I were having breakfast one morning in Medellín, I started talking about a trip to Japan I was planning. Angie was full of curiosity, so I went upstairs and bought her a ticket to Tokyo. I told her she could pay me back whenever.

Angie's been to more than fifty countries since then. Japan's still her favorite.

I told Mike that it would probably be just Angie and me traveling. Mike was about twenty years older than Angie, but they got on very well. They made each other laugh. And Mike preferred to travel with a small group. Some of the trips I'd taken got kind of big; we were like a traveling circus, and I was the ringmaster. Not Mike's scene.

"I'll think about it," said Mike. "It sounds awesome."

"Don't think too long, Mike," I said. "The pandemic won't last. This is our chance."

MARCH 2020

I never bought those plane tickets to Angola. We were still debating whether to go when, at the beginning of March, fears about the virus surged. All of a sudden, it was the only thing anyone talked about. So we decided to wait.

On March 1, Andrew Cuomo, the governor of New York, announced the state's first case of the novel coronavirus. A guy in Westchester had tested positive, as had a group of people he'd been in contact with.

New Yorkers reacted to the news by panic-buying. They bought rice, pasta, toilet paper. They bought hand sanitizer and surgical masks. But they still went out to restaurants and theaters and bars. Looking back, I think a lot of people probably caught the virus as they stood in line at stores to buy products they wouldn't need or squeezed into crowded restaurants for brunch.

All the same, the world was on high alert. The stock market tanked, and oil prices fell. On March 11, Tedros Adhanom Ghebreyesus, director general of the World Health Organization, declared the first global pandemic caused by a coronavirus. Italy locked down, then France and Spain.

At work, we wondered what New York City would do. Would the mayor close the schools? Would people be confined to their homes? Would the subway shut down?

Some of the EMTs and paramedics dismissed the dangers, said that people were being hysterical. But Stephen Northmore, a paramedic at Station 40—very serious, very disciplined—was grim. He'd been talking to some EMTs who were laughing off the virus. "Are you ready for the shitstorm that's coming?" he'd asked them. "Are you ready to be the only people on the street other than the National Guard?"

Then we heard that an EMT at a station in Coney Island had tested positive. His girlfriend was a flight attendant and she'd tested positive too. The assumption was that she had infected him. The EMT had worked on an ambulance with five other EMTs over the course of the week before his positive test. He had been shut up in an ambulance with them for hours on end. It seemed extremely likely that they had caught the virus too.

FDNY EMS asked those five EMTs to self-quarantine for fourteen days, meaning that they should isolate in their homes. The department said it was tracking eleven patients who had had contact with the EMT. But the department had no way to test its members. If EMS workers wanted to know if they'd caught the virus, they had to go and line up at the hospitals with everybody else. The idea of screening EMS workers—testing them regularly to make sure they weren't spreading the virus—was a pie-in-the-sky dream.

On March 15, Mayor Bill de Blasio said that New York City's schools would close immediately. Then restaurants, nightclubs, theaters, bars. A day earlier, Cuomo had announced the state's first COVID-19 death. The deceased was an eighty-two-year-old woman who'd suffered from emphysema, a lung condition in which the alveoli, the tiny sacs that collect air, are damaged. It seemed that any kind of underlying issue affecting the lungs made a patient more vulnerable to the virus.

The mayor then rushed to his beloved YMCA in Park Slope to squeeze in one last fitness session. He should have been working flat out to help the city prepare for what was coming. Getting the PPE that was needed to all the frontline workers. But his spokesperson said that he wanted to do something that kept him "grounded." As if doing bench presses would increase his leadership skills.

And leadership was sorely needed. With the news of New York's first documented COVID-19 fatality, the mood in the city suddenly shifted. It was as if the pandemic had snuck in while we were sleeping, and we'd woken up to find it looming over the bed. Panic-buying became plain old panic.

It didn't help that the mayor was hopelessly out of step with the pace of the virus and the science of how it spread. For the first two weeks of March, he'd dismissed the dangers. He'd told New Yorkers, "Go about your lives, go about your business." He'd offered movie recommendations (specifically, an aptly named Italian crime drama called *The Traitor*).

The mayor made one misleading statement after the next. To be infected by the coronavirus, the mayor told an interviewer on MSNBC on March 5, you needed to have "the kind of exposure that you wouldn't get on the subway." Coronavirus wouldn't spread in a stadium or at a conference, he said a few days later. It would spread only among people who were "close up to each other."

Just a few days before he closed the largest school system in the country, de Blasio said that mass school closures were not on the menu. It was something that could happen in theory, he said, but was it "anywhere near to where we are now? No."

He'd soon be eating his words.

On March 17, one day after the city's schools closed, I stood in an apartment in Sunset Park with a man who was having trouble breathing. The man lay on a reclining chair in the living room of a one-bedroom apartment. There were white curtains in the window tied back with a loop of cloth. The patient was Puerto Rican, fifty-two years old. Not very tall. His skin was the color of light coffee, and his thick hair wasn't yet gray.

"I don't feel right," he said.

It was St. Patrick's Day. But for the first time in more than two hundred years, there would be no parade in New York. Or Boston. Or Chicago. Or even Dublin.

The day before, the number of confirmed cases of COVID-19 in New York City had risen to 923, and a quarter of them were in Brooklyn. The total had more or less doubled in twenty-four hours and had almost doubled in the twenty-four hours before that. So far, according to the city's official count, ten people had died of the virus. The writing had been on the wall for weeks, but now we could finally read it.

The Sunset Park call came over as a diff breather, a patient having trouble breathing. That could mean anything from pneumonia to flu to asthma. The call type wasn't fever/cough. I put on a surgical mask and gloves, as always. Nothing out of the ordinary in terms of protection.

A paramedic crew arrived at the man's apartment just as I did. They were from Lutheran Hospital in nearby Bay Ridge. The medic who was teching—taking the lead on patient care—sat down next to the man. (In EMS jargon, the paramedic who is in the back of the ambulance with the patient is *teching*, and the paramedic who is driving the bus is *wrecking*. As in "wrecking the vehicle." But when the wreckers aren't driving, they assist with patient care.)

The patient told the medic that he had a headache. He massaged his forehead with his fingers. Then he tapped his chest. "I can't catch my breath."

"Sir, how long have you been feeling this way?" the medic asked. "Are you experiencing any chest pain?"

"A few days, I haven't felt good," the guy said. "Chest pain? No. Just I find it hard to breathe."

"Don't worry. We're going to take care of you. We're just going to take some vitals. Do you have any medical problems?"

"No."

"When did you last see a physician?"

"I don't know. It's been a while."

"Okay, sir. Let's take a look at you."

The medic checked the guy's pulse. It was over 100 beats per minute. A normal resting heart rate is usually around 60 to 80 beats per minute. His blood pressure was 150/90. Probably some kind of flu or a chest infection, I figured. Maybe pneumonia.

"Let's see what he's satting," I said.

The medic fished in his bag for a pulse oximeter. A small device that clips onto the end of your finger, it measures the level of oxygen saturation in your blood by sending beams of red and infrared light through your fingertip to a sensor on the other side. The sensor reads how much of each kind of light is absorbed and uses that to calculate the oxygen saturation level of your blood. If your blood is well oxygenated, it absorbs more of the infrared light and less of the red light. If your blood is low in oxygen, it absorbs more of the red light and less of the infrared light.

In healthy patients, the pulse oximeter should read 95 percent or higher. In patients who have bad asthma or congestive heart failure, the reading might drop to 80 percent. These patients won't be talking. They will be concentrating on breathing. They will be struggling. They might by cyanotic, meaning their lips or fingertips are blue because of the lack of oxygen in their blood. They will be gasping and using accessory muscles such as back muscles to try to pull more air into their lungs.

The reading from our patient was 74 percent.

"Wait. Let's test him again," I said. The reading didn't make sense. The patient was talking in full sentences. He was not cyanotic. He was not gasping. He looked a little uncomfortable, and his heart rate was elevated. But that was all. The EMT took off the pulse ox, warmed up the guy's finger to make sure his blood was circulating properly, and put the device back on.

Now it read 72 percent.

"Wow. It must be broken," I said. "Let's try another one. Do we have another pulse ox?"

"I've got one, Lou," the second medic said. "This definitely works," he added. "I calibrated it this morning."

"Cool. Let's try yours."

The medic got his bag. Dug around for the pulse oximeter. Put it on the guy's finger. The patient was quiet. He seemed focused on his breathing.

The monitor read 70 percent.

Shit. Something strange was going on. Something serious. The symptoms didn't add up. But this was bad.

The medic listened to the man's lungs. "I can hear the air moving," he said. "But it sounds far away."

I understood what he meant. When you listen to a healthy person taking a deep breath, you hear a sound like air rushing into a balloon. This man's lungs sounded a bit hollow, like when you knock on an empty pipe. We put a nonrebreather mask on him—a mask with a one-way valve that allowed him to breathe in air with a high concentration of oxygen and exhale air into the room—and set the oxygen flow to ten liters per minute.

"Let's go," I said. "Let's get him down to the bus."

We'd been with the man for about fifteen minutes. Since we'd arrived, he had become dangerously hypoxic, meaning that the tissues of his body were not receiving enough oxygen. The reason for this wasn't clear, but perhaps he had heart failure, I thought. Whatever the cause, if we couldn't increase the oxygen level in his blood, he could die.

The medics bundled the man into the stair chair. We wrapped him in a sheet and carried him down the two flights of stairs to the street. We put an IV in so that we could give him medication quickly if he needed it. We put the pulse oximeter on his fingertip one more time.

He was down to 60 percent. Jesus. It was a miracle that he was conscious. I couldn't figure out how he'd been able to talk to us just a few minutes ago.

The crew loaded the patient into the ambulance and drove off to Lutheran Hospital.

I bumped into the two paramedics later that day. "How'd that guy do?" I said. "The one whose saturation was really low?"

"Sunset Park?" one of the medics said. "Lou, he coded. He coded just as we were arriving at the hospital. We couldn't get him back."

The Puerto Rican patient was my Patient Zero. I'm fairly sure that I'd treated someone with coronavirus before that day. Probably several people. But that patient's case was the first one that I can look back on and say with certainty, "That was COVID." He hadn't been tested—he might never make it into the official case count—but he had it. In retrospect, his symptoms were unmistakable.

Over the weeks that followed, the ways that COVID presented became all too familiar. Patients had unbelievably low oxygen saturation levels. Blue lips. They'd felt poorly one day and could barely breathe the next. Many patients who called an ambulance were dead before we reached them.

EMS workers' understanding of COVID-19 was extremely limited. We weren't sure how it spread. How it attacked the body. We learned as we went along, comparing notes with one another, talking to emergency department nurses and doctors. We were all feeling our way forward.

Most patients suffered some kind of respiratory illness with a spiking fever and a dry cough. Some patients described feeling "like an elephant is sitting on my chest." They talked about shortness of breath. In X-rays taken at the hospital, their lungs often looked opaque, as if they were filled with ground glass.

If patients we were treating were having trouble breathing, we gave them supplemental oxygen from a portable tank that we carried on the ambulance. We placed nonrebreather masks over their faces. If someone couldn't breathe at all, we sedated and intubated him or her, then hooked up a bag to oxygen and manually ventilated the patient.

In the hospital, those patients would be transferred to mechanical ventilators.

We also started to recognize the other telltale symptoms of COVID-19: a loss of taste or smell, headaches, body aches much like those experienced with the flu, diarrhea, conjunctivitis, and rashes. In serious cases, the body's inflammatory response to infection from SARS-CoV-2 was so extreme that it damaged the patient's kidneys, liver, heart, and lungs.

We also learned that the virus caused tiny blood clots—or emboli—in the lungs that led to the blood becoming poorly oxygenated. That meant that a patient who appeared to be breathing without difficulty might not be effectively transferring oxygen into the bloodstream. Patients might be able to talk but still have dangerously low levels of oxygen saturation. Like my Patient Zero. He probably had emboli in his lungs, but that possibility never crossed my mind. We were groping around in the dark for clues about the disease and the virus that caused it.

Around St. Patrick's Day, the day of my Patient Zero, I noticed many more fever/cough calls coming over the radio. The computer-aided Dispatch screen in my office—the screen where I track 911 calls and the ambulances responding to them—began to fill with calls that carried the letters *FC*.

Bones told me that one night, he called in a notification to Brookdale University Hospital Medical Center in Brooklyn that he was bringing in a fever/cough patient. That was the protocol—consult with telemetry and then notify the hospital that you're on your way with a suspected COVID case.

After he alerted the hospital, Bones kept the radio open for the rest of the drive, which took about seven minutes, he said. He listened to dozens of other units around Brooklyn notifying different hospitals that they were transporting patients. They shared a single call type:

Fever/cough.

Fever/cough.

Fever/cough, fever/cough, fever/cough.

At the hospital, Bones turned to his partner. "Jeez, you hear that?" he said. "It's like, 'Houston, we have a problem.'"

Picture this: An EMS station in New York City. It's a morning in early spring 2020. Outside the station, there's a big truck. It's full of boxes. The doors to the station are open. Smiling EMS workers unload the boxes from the truck. They pass them hand to hand in a line. An EMS lieutenant ticks off items on a list. Another member directs the boxes to the storage area downstairs. The boxes contain N95 masks of all sizes, gowns, gloves, face shields. Cots so that service members can sleep at the station if they need to. Pillows, blankets. Microwavable meals. Washing machines so they can launder contaminated uniforms.

In the middle of all the activity, Lillian Bonsignore, the EMS chief, arrives. She climbs onto the step of an ambulance that's parked outside the station. The members gather around. She delivers a rousing speech: "We're facing the unknown. It's going to be hard. But we've got your backs. We are all in this together. And remember," she says, "we're New York's Best!"

That would have been a heartening scene, right? Like a rousing movie sequence in which whistling soldiers set up camp in preparation for war.

Sadly, it never happened.

There was no truck bursting with supplies. There was no visit from the EMS chief. There was no line of cheerful EMTs. The fire department continued to send buck slips—internal memos about which mask to wear and when to wear it, what PPE to use, how to triage a suspected COVID case. But they provided little in the way of supplies. And less in the way of moral support.

To be fair, a couple of stations did receive washing machines.

With little guidance from the higher-ups, we'd tried to handle the preparations ourselves. During the first week of March, I'd gone down into the basement of Station 40 with Bones to look at our stocks of masks and gowns. Bones was in charge of keeping track of basic life support supplies for the station. The basement was stacked with BLS materials: four-inch-square gauze bandages used for most wounds; neck braces; stair chairs; oropharyngeal airways (hook-shaped tubes used to keep patients' airways open); sterile water for washing wounds; cold packs; obstetrical kits (infant swaddle, placenta bag); urinals; plastic tubs for stowing needles and other sharps. There was a box of red felt Christmas stockings, each decorated with a member's name. A plastic Christmas tree.

Bones and I counted the boxes of N95 masks. There were half a dozen—that added up to a few hundred masks.

That was nothing out of the ordinary. In normal times, very few people wore masks of any kind. If you had a patient who was coughing or vomiting, you'd wear a surgical mask, one of the blue and white ones that New Yorkers snapped up during the early days of the pandemic. Those we had boxes and boxes of.

Surgical masks are made of polypropylene, a nonwoven papery substance that allows air to pass through it but not droplets of moisture. So if you're wearing a surgical mask and somebody sprays blood on you, the mask will catch those droplets. It protects against droplets better than a cloth mask does, because cloth masks are made of woven fibers and are therefore more permeable. Still, the surgical masks are loose-fitting. They don't stop airborne particles from passing into your nose and mouth. For that, you need an N95.

The N95 mask is designed to filter out 95 percent of airborne particles with a diameter of 0.3 microns or greater. The mask is supposed to fit snugly, so that there's a seal around your face. That's why the fire department fits everyone for the mask once a year. Before the pandemic, the masks were reserved for when you were dealing with suspected cases of certain infectious diseases, like tuberculosis. Everyone in the station kept a few in the correct size on the ambulance. The spares sat on a shelf in the basement.

Now we needed more. A lot more. The stocks we had would last a week, maybe two. Judging by what had happened in China and Italy, the pandemic was going to be going on a hell of a lot longer than that.

We weren't the only service that lacked PPE. Every frontline worker in the city was struggling—nurses, doctors, police, subway drivers, and station agents. Amid the run on masks, some public workers were even told by their organizations that they didn't need them. A memo issued by the Metropolitan Transport Authority, which runs the subway, instructed employees not to wear masks to work because they "will not help," and wearing them might contribute to panic-buying. For dozens of employees, the rules amounted to a death sentence.

Bones had sent a request for N95 masks to the FDNY Incident Management Team, the unit that oversees large-scale incidents and emergencies such as hurricanes and earthquakes. We figured they'd drop off masks, gowns, gloves, disinfectant wipes for cleaning the ambulance. But days went by. Eventually, IMT sent a box of surgical masks and a couple of boxes of N95s. Nothing else.

About a week after I treated the Puerto Rican man on St. Patrick's Day, my protective gown split during another call in Sunset Park. At this point, EMTs and paramedics were wearing gowns, gloves, and N95s on every call. The gowns were flimsy. Some looked like the bibs worn by the ladies who served lunch at my elementary school. Some were so small, they seemed like they were made for children. It was like wearing a large paper napkin. The sleeves tore as you put your arms in. The ties at the back snapped off as you tried to tie them. We would arrive at the scene of a cardiac arrest, pull on a gown, and begin CPR, and the gown would fall apart.

The patient in Sunset Park was a middle-aged man. He was in terrible shape, feverish and vomiting. The apartment was small. The patient's family stood in the living room. They looked alarmed. By now, I knew the signs of COVID infection. I looked at the family's faces, one after another. They were pale and clammy. *They have COVID too,* I thought. The apartment was probably teeming with the virus.

I went back to the command vehicle. My gown and uniform were spattered with vomit. I felt like I had coronavirus crawling over my pants, my shirt, as if I'd been sprinkled with the virus. I opened the back of the SUV, peeled off the gown, and put it into a red bag for hazardous waste. Then I unbuttoned my shirt and stripped down to my T-shirt in the street. I had a clean shirt in the back of the truck. I took off my mask, held the mask with my gloved hand, removed the glove, and folded the mask inside it. Put it in the red bag. It was a routine I would repeat, day in and day out, for months.

New York had become a ghost town. Shops were closed. Kids stayed home from school. Even the playgrounds were locked.

Horse racing was suspended. I'd worked one final shift at Aqueduct the week before things began to shut down. There were races, but no spectators. The place was more desolate than ever. I wondered how Sam—the old man I treated there in February—was doing. His beloved racetrack was off-limits now. What did he do to pass the time?

While most of the city had shut down, its hospitals were on a war footing. They suited up their medical staffs in whatever protective gear they could get their hands on. Canceled surgeries to keep the number of patients down.

My own surgery had just been pushed back till May, at least. I wondered how long it would be, realistically, before it was rescheduled. I worried that the surgeon wouldn't be able to salvage my tendon and that I'd have to receive a graft from a cadaver, which would make the recovery period longer and mean that I would regain less motion and strength. Normally, to make sure the torn tendon is sufficiently elastic, surgeons perform the procedure within a couple of months of the injury. I had waited five months and counting. I regretted not having gotten my arm fixed when I could, but how could I have known what was going to happen?

Emergency departments were quickly being modified to deal with the influx of virus patients. Maimonides Medical Center erected a tent outside and started triaging patients there. The hospital had two emergency areas. It separated suspected COVID-19 patients from non-COVID patients. Brooklyn Hospital Center in Fort Greene also set up a triage tent on the street. They screened walk-in patients before they entered the building. Inside the emergency area, they built a wall to separate non-COVID patients from patients who appeared to be infected. Everybody was improvising.

I ran into the station one day to take a bathroom break and saw Bill Keating, one of our EMTs, who'd just dropped a patient at University Hospital in Crown Heights, a public hospital that's part of the SUNY Downstate Health Sciences University.

Keating told me that when he rolled the patient into the emergency department, he saw nurses in white isolation suits: hoods, face shields, masks.

"It was like the scene in *ET* when the alien is sick and the people are walking around in hazmat gear," Keating said. "I thought, *Holy shit, this is real.*"

Not long after New York City shut down, a lot of its residents got sick. By March 31, the city had recorded a total of 41,771 cases of COVID—an increase of almost 4,500 percent from the tally of 923 that was published the day that I met my Patient Zero. And that was with a very limited testing infrastructure; the true number of infections was likely many times higher.

Many of the sick were dying. The city went from recording two or three deaths related to COVID each day in mid-March to more than four hundred a day at the end of the month. By March 31, the city said, 8,549 people had been hospitalized with the virus and 1,096 had died (a figure that, we later learned, vastly underestimated the real toll). It felt like a bomb had gone off.

On a normal day in a normal year, the volume of medical calls to 911 in New York City is around 4,000. On September 11, 2001, that number rose to 6,500. Many of those calls were panicked people reporting the same thing. During the last week of March 2020, the volume of daily calls rose to 5,200 and then to over 7,000.

March 30, 2020, was the busiest day in the history of the Fire Department of New York's emergency medical service. We received 7,253 calls. That's one call every twelve seconds. EMTs called for backup from paramedic crews and were told that the nearest available crew was on the other side of Brooklyn or in Manhattan.

Many of the coronavirus protocols that we had been told to follow—taking ambulances out of service to disinfect them, isolating at home for fourteen days if we'd been exposed to someone with COVID—went out the window. They just weren't practical. They were designed for an epidemic that involved a trickle of contagious patients, like the Ebola patient Mike transferred to Bellevue back in 2014. They weren't designed for a deluge of patients that filled up every ICU in the city.

And a deluge was what we faced. New York City's medical pipeline was close to bursting. That pipeline began on the ambulance, ran through hospitals' emergency departments and ICUs, and, for too many patients, ended on a refrigerated truck. Whether they wound up there due to COVID or because of some other condition, the root cause of death was often the same: the city's health-care system had all but collapsed.

EMTs and medics were transferring patients to emergency departments filled with infected New Yorkers in hospitals that had no beds. Patients were dying in those crowded hospitals and being shipped to temporary morgues. In a city where people normally had to fight for a parking spot or a subway seat, the streets were empty. But the medical system was jammed like never before, and it was costing lives.

By the last week of March, many emergency departments were so swamped with patients that they directed ambulances to go to other facilities—what's called going on diversion. As soon as one hospital came back online, a different hospital went on diversion.

These teeming EDs became a bottleneck for EMS crews, who waited far longer than normal to transfer patients. One of the EMTs from Station 40 waited an hour while the hospital wrangled a gurney for his patient, who was breathing on a ventilator; there was literally nowhere to put him.

Crews with patients who were so sick that they'd normally be rushed straight through the doors were waiting in line for ninety minutes.

The last week of March, Ciro Napolitano, an EMT from Station 40, stepped into the triage area of a hospital in Brooklyn's Midwood neighborhood to find a line of EMS units waiting to transfer patients. Ciro was in his twenties, from Bensonhurst, the neighborhood where Joe Cengiz had lived. Very chatty.

Every patient on the line looked like death, Ciro told me. Pale. Gasping.

The ambulance crews stared at Ciro. Their eyes said, *Not another one.*

Ciro had notified the hospital about his patient because the man's oxygen saturation level was in the fifties. "Sorry, guys," Ciro said. "I called in a note. I have to go ahead."

On his way in, Ciro waved to an EMT in the line. She worked in Coney Island. The EMT looked burned out. Her patient was semiconscious, very sick-looking.

Ten minutes later, Ciro walked out to find the Coney Island EMT pumping the man's chest. The patient had gone into cardiac arrest right there in the entrance to the emergency department. They had been waiting in line for that long.

That day or the next, Keating pulled up at a different hospital in Midwood. The emergency department staff were rushing back and forth. They seemed to be down to two or three nurses.

Bill gave the triage nurse the patient assessment. As the nurse punched the patient's information into the computer, Bill leaned over to his partner.

"I'd still take this ER over that other one any day of the week," he said, referring to another Brooklyn South hospital. The staff there had a reputation for being rude. Probably because they were always over-worked.

The nurse looked up at Keating. "Don't bring anyone else here," she said. Her voice trembled. "We have only two or three nurses. We're on diversion."

She looked as if she was going to cry. "Half of us are sick," she said. "One of us is on a vent upstairs."

Keating swallowed and looked away. There was nothing he could say. He knew he'd be back soon with another patient.

"Please," the nurse said. "Don't bring anyone else."

And the emergency departments weren't the only bottlenecks. With FDNY ambulance crews picking up hundreds of COVID patients every day, the telemetry office couldn't keep up. There was only one physician fielding all the questions from our crews. One doctor for the whole of EMS in a city of over eight million people. It was chaos.

Around the time that the city locked down, Stephen Northmore—the paramedic who had warned the unconcerned EMTs about the looming apocalypse—picked up a patient who was sweating bullets and coughing up yellowish-green sputum. His oxygen saturation was not that low, but he had other symptoms of coronavirus infection.

Northmore called telemetry to ask which hospital he should transfer the patient to. He was on the line for fifty-two minutes. The para-medics who were in the telemetry office fielding calls—taking down preliminary information on the patient and proposed treatment—said that they had thirteen other units on hold. They were all waiting to consult with one doctor.

So Northmore and his partner spent the better part of an hour in a very tight space with a patient who was coughing up gunk and presumably had COVID. In the end, the medic at the other end of the phone told Northmore to head to Brookdale because it was closest. He never got an answer from the doctor.

Soon after this, FDNY told us not to call telemetry anymore, just head to the nearest hospital and pray that it had the capacity to take one more patient. All bets were off.

It wasn't just that there weren't enough beds and nurses and telemetry doctors. The PPE supply crunch, too, was almost immediate. There was a worldwide shortage. Everybody everywhere was scrambling for masks and gowns and disinfectant. Paramedics swiped antiseptic wipes from emergency rooms so they could clean their ambulances. They brought Lysol from home. EMTs from hospital ambulance units and volunteer units tried to scrounge masks from us. Given the shortage of N95s, medical personnel were wearing KN95s—the Chinese version of the N95, which offered very similar protection—construction masks, knockoff N95s, doubled-up surgical masks. Whatever they could get.

I was working on a nursing-home call in late March with a medic from one of the Brooklyn South hospitals. She wore a blue face covering that looked like a construction worker's mask. She asked me if I could spare a mask. She looked like she felt a little awkward, as if she were asking for money. Some days I did have an extra mask and I had no problem parting with it. But on that day, I had nothing to give her. Her face fell.

The FDNY had a better supply of masks than most of the private ambulance fleets, but we were still running low. Every government agency was competing for suddenly vital resources like these. The United States has about four thousand nuclear warheads, but apparently, nobody in government thought to keep a stockpile of dollar-twenty-five masks. And now Donald Trump had states competing with one another for PPE and hospital supplies, making their own deals with China.

FDNY told its members to use N95s only when they were treating patients with suspected COVID-19 or when they needed to perform procedures that might cause aerosolization—that is, procedures that might make the patient spray tiny coronavirus-infected droplets all over your eyes and mouth.

One such procedure was intubation, which was becoming increasingly routine, since COVID destroyed people's lungs. To intubate a patient, you have to lean right over his gaping mouth. You have to sweep the tongue aside with a special blade and look for the vocal cords. You have to thread a tube between the cords. You're close enough to the patient to count his fillings. There's no way you're not going to get spittle and mucus flying at you. And if you weren't wearing a mask, there was little chance you'd avoid catching the virus.

On top of restricting the use of N95s, the FDNY asked EMS members to keep track of the N95s they used. Imagine: You're tearing around the city, trying to protect yourself from a potentially deadly virus, and at the end of the day you have to fill out paperwork to justify your decision to use a mask? How petty and wrongheaded could you get? There was no way I was going to play along. If an EMT or medic came to me asking for a mask, that person got a mask. No questions asked.

As if we needed proof of the lack of adequate PPE, EMTs and paramedics all over the city began to fall sick.

A few days after the patient died on the line for the emergency department, Ciro came down with COVID. Then Kenny. And Bones's wife, an EMS lieutenant in Brownsville. She was asthmatic, so she had real trouble breathing.

For two weeks, every day, Bones went to work in the most dangerous environment that any of us had ever known, then rushed home, shopped, took care of his wife, his eighteen-month-old daughter, and his two stepsons, then raced back to the station to start the cycle all over again.

At the end of March, there was no dedicated testing facility for EMS workers. Even eighteen months later, at the time of this writing, there is still no such thing. One paramedic drove out to a pop-up testing site—like the one established at Aqueduct, where I worked before the pandemic—and waited hours, only to be turned away because they'd run out of tests. The city was consistently touting testing as the key to fighting the virus, yet it couldn't even test the people on the front lines of that fight.

Ciro, Kenny, and Bones's wife—as sick as they were—endured the virus and recovered at home. That would be true of many members who became ill in March and April.

Juan Rios, however, was not so lucky. Juan caught COVID and ended up in the hospital.

Juan was an EMT at Station 40. Been on the job for years. Juan was thirty-nine years old in the spring of 2020. He went home early one night feeling shaky and feverish. He developed a hacking cough. For a few days, he monitored his oxygen saturation at home. He used a mask to give himself supplemental oxygen.

But after a few days, Juan was running out of oxygen supplies. He could barely walk. So he called 911.

When I heard that Juan was in the hospital, I was worried. And I was furious. Juan's being hospitalized drove home how much danger EMS workers faced and how little the department seemed to value our lives. We'd been left to battle it out on the empty streets without proper protection. We were expected to risk everything, but nobody seemed to care too much about trying to keep us safe.

The top brass of EMS—Chief Bonsignore, Assistant Chiefs Alvin Suriel and Jonathan Pistilli—were in the wind. I thought we would at least get a visit from one or two of them, that they would swing by the station with bagels and ask what we needed, but no. By contrast, Dinorah Claudio, the chief of Division 5 (my division), went station to station to ask what supplies we needed, then tried to wrangle them for us; she called to check on members who were sick. Medics in the

Bronx said that Michael Fields, a division chief, went to the local hospitals to help out crews and speed up patient transfers. But since calls had started clogging up 911 in mid-March, the most senior chiefs had been working from home. They were nowhere to be seen.

We were starting to notice that the virus didn't affect all New Yorkers equally. White-collar workers could—and did—work from home, and affluent people escaped to houses upstate, but supermarket employees and bus drivers and delivery people had to stay and run the risk of infection, often without protective gear. That split should not have been mirrored in the hierarchy at EMS. We were an essential service. We were a team. Weren't we?

Juan, who was now wheezing in a bed in the intensive care unit at Lutheran Hospital, was not allowed to have visitors. But that didn't stop Bones. Late one night, Bones snuck past the guards at Lutheran and ran up the back stairs to see his friend. Bones knew that he would be in deep shit if he was caught. But he wasn't easily scared. He'd worked on 9/11. Juan had told Bones he wanted a Pepsi and some chips, and Bones was going to make sure he got them.

"Someone had to have the balls to do it," he said. And besides, Bones had his broccoli rabe virus protection.

Bones crept down the corridor. It was creepy. The nurses were cloaked in long gowns, goggles, face shields. Juan was in a dim room, loudly pulling air into his lungs. Bones's heart dropped at the sight of him.

"Hey, Bones," Juan said. He could barely speak. "This thing is really kicking my ass."

Bones put the chips and the soda by the bed. He told Juan that everyone at the station was rooting for him. Then he left.

Looking back, he said, "I felt like I was taking a prisoner his last meal."

More members fell sick: Jimmy Mac. Harney. Bove, Cekic. Petrizzo, Finkel, Scala. Incorvaia, Birdman, Polizzi, Don. So many members were out sick that the department called in retired EMTs and paramedics and took the paramedics who'd been working desk jobs and put them on ambulances. If the EMT or paramedic who was supposed to relieve you after your tour didn't show, you had to stay.

To deal with the shortage of crews, the department relaxed the regulations about who should staff the ambulances. Normally, a paramedic rides the bus with another paramedic, and an EMT rides with another EMT. Now, a paramedic could ride with an EMT, and an EMT could ride with a firefighter—not that I remember that ever happening. The fire department had issued an order on March 7 instructing firefighters not to respond to fever/cough medical calls. Firefighters would still go to critical calls like cardiac arrests, the department said. But if a call came over as fever/cough, firefighters wouldn't respond. The department wanted them to stay behind the lines.

In an effort to protect their families, EMS workers all over the city were sleeping on the couches or in the rec rooms at their stations or in their cars. A friend of mine, David Timothy, a dispatcher, usually worked one week in New York and then spent the next week in Chicago with his family. He flew from Chicago to New York on an eerily empty flight on March 14 and didn't see his eight-year-old twins again until July.

I lived alone, so I didn't face that dilemma. Still, COVID made us all nervous. Every time I arrived home after a tour, I peeled off my clothes as soon as I closed the front door and put everything in a bag to take to the laundromat. Then I jumped in the shower. At work, I wiped down the entire command vehicle before my tour: the radio, the dials, the steering wheel, the dashboard, the MDT (mobile data terminal), the door handles, the oxygen tanks. Everything. I saw what the virus did to people. I couldn't avoid being exposed to the virus in people's homes or in the station. But in my vehicle, at least, I did what I could.

I was mainly on the road during those weeks. Lieutenants normally alternate between being in the field and sitting the desk. But I wanted to be with the crews and patients, and my fellow lieutenants seemed okay with being at the station. My injury meant that I shouldn't lift people unless there was no alternative. This I found out the hard way one day in March, when I tried to help an EMT lift a patient in a stair chair. I grabbed the front of the chair and felt a bolt of pain in my elbow. My arm became weak, as if the muscles were giving way, then began to tingle.

Lifting aside, though, I could do my job—helping supervise patient care, dealing with difficult situations, pronouncing patients who had died. So I stuck to the road.

Now and then, I did work a tour at the station. And from my office one night, I watched the city collapse.

It was around eleven o'clock. The radio had been barking nonstop. Assignments poured in. The computer-aided Dispatch screen showed dozens of 911 calls on hold in each borough. Dozens of people waiting for an ambulance.

Normally, a call comes in and we assign a unit immediately. It's rare to have calls on hold. On a crazy day—Hurricane Sandy, a heat wave—we might run short of ambulances and start shifting them from other parts of the city. But not for a long period.

On this night, there were calls holding for two hours, three hours. One patient in Queens had been waiting for six. Since that patient had called, two thousand other calls had come in.

I stared at the screen in horror. *Look at all those people,* I thought. *Hundreds of New Yorkers who can't get an ambulance. Which of those callers is having a heart attack? Which of those callers is having a stroke? Who's going to die before we can get to them?* We had people with respiratory problems waiting on hold for an hour. As for less urgent calls—a grandma with dehydration; a person with a bad stomachache—there was a chance that they'd be on hold forever; that we might never make it down the list to them. If you broke your ankle in New York City in late March 2020, you would have had to hop to the hospital. And once you got there, you might have had to set the bone yourself.

. . .

By the last week of March, New York City had become the epicenter of coronavirus infection in the United States. New York State at that moment accounted for almost half of all infections in America, and most of those cases were in the five boroughs that made up the state's largest city. Hospitals didn't have enough ventilators or continuous positive airway pressure (CPAP) machines, which use mild pressure to keep a patient's airways open and ease breathing. They didn't have enough gowns or N95 masks. They didn't have enough staff.

In a city of hospitals that were at the breaking point, NYC Health and Hospitals/Elmhurst was one of the worst hit. It's a big public hospital built in the 1950s in Queens. Around the hospital are low-income neighborhoods that are home to legions of essential workers from all over the world: Colombia, India, Nepal, Bangladesh, Mexico, China, the Philippines. It's a true melting pot. But during the pandemic, the area became a death trap. Woodside, Corona, Jackson Heights, East Elmhurst—these neighborhoods suffered more than almost any others in New York City. The official death rate in these neighborhoods was three or four times that of wealthy sections of Manhattan.

Elmhurst had become the epicenter of the epicenter. The situation in the hospital made headlines on March 25. That day, the *New York Times* published a video filmed by an Elmhurst ER doctor. In a shaking voice, she talked about how unprepared they were, about how the hospital was barely coping, about how they were trying to get more ventilators. Officials kept saying that things would be fine. But they wouldn't be fine, the doctor said.

The next day, I got a call from a lieutenant at Station 46, which is next to Elmhurst Hospital. The lieutenant knew that I was trying to get the media interested in the situation facing EMS. It was frustrating to see news reports about how tough things were inside the hospitals but not about how tough things were on the street. I'm pretty active on Twitter, so I'd been tweeting about de Blasio never mentioning us when he talked about first responders. I'd been begging for more PPE. And I'd been begging people on Twitter to stay home and keep safe. I'd tweeted @NYCMayorsOffice, @nytimes, @CNN. I'd retweeted messages of support from Andrew Gounardes, the state senator representing New York's Twenty-Second District—southern Brooklyn.

"Anthony, there's a ton of television crews outside the hospital," the lieutenant said. "Dozens. You should come down. This is your chance."

It was my day off. I was free. I could go and speak to the media as union vice president.

I called Mike Greco, the vice president of Local 2507. His union represents uniformed EMTs, paramedics, and fire inspectors. My union represents the officers—lieutenants and captains. I told him we had an opportunity to spread the word about the plight of our union members.

"Let's go," he said.

Elmhurst was a madhouse. A long line of people snaked up a ramp behind police barricades. They were waiting to be tested in a white tent that had been erected outside, next to the emergency area. Some of the people had waited hours and hours. Huge, smiling faces of children looked down at them from a mural on the side of the hospital. There were ambulances lined up at the entrance to the trauma center, waiting to drop patients. The hospital was now a symbol of the collapse of the health system: So many patients. Not enough testing. Not enough PPE. Not enough medical workers.

Outside the entrance of the emergency department, there was a phalanx of television cameras. It was like a red carpet for emergency medical workers, except that the gowns were made of yellow paper and the award was an unused N95 mask or a slice of pizza.

I approached the bank of camera crews. I didn't know where to start. I'm not a shy person, but this was new to me.

Okay, Anthony, I thought. *Just pick a camera.*

I walked up to the closest crew. They were from Agence France-Presse. Pronounced "Ajonse Fronse-Press." I know that now. It's a huge news agency, but I didn't know anything about it then. There was a female journalist. I introduced myself. "I'm Anthony Almojera," I said. "I'm vice president of the EMS officers' union. And I have a story to tell you."

That was it. After the first interview, Mike peeled off. I walked down the line, introducing myself to each news crew.

"What you're seeing on TV is not the whole story," I said. "There's another story out there. And it involves EMS."

What was going on in the hospitals was also going on in the ambulances, I said. And for all the people who were dying in the hospital, many were dying before they even got there. In EMS, we saw this: People dying in their homes. In our ambulances. In the slow lines to get into the emergency departments. The numbers being published by the government didn't take those people into account, I said.

The official death toll was frightening. The real death toll was far worse.

By the time I moved to the third news crew, there were crews from other media outlets waiting to speak to me. Channel 4, Channel 11, the BBC, CNN. Univision. The *Daily News*. I was on fire. For the first time in days, I felt like something I was doing was making a difference. I told the news reporters how the lack of supplies inside the hospitals was mirrored in EMS, about how four hundred members were out sick with suspected cases of coronavirus and how the rest were run ragged.

A couple of days later, I drove up to Yonkers to see Mike Sullivan. I had a couple of television interviews to do using video apps like Zoom, and Mike was going to help me look as professional as possible.

At the time, Mike coordinated the FDNY's advanced-life-support operations in the Bronx—he managed all the paramedic crews and kept track of supplies and training.

But what I needed at that moment was not Mike the Medic; I needed Mike the Actor.

Mike had a basic setup at home for recording auditions: a tripod and a ring light, a plain backdrop. He'd suggested that I come over to his apartment to do the interviews; he would make me look like I knew what I was doing.

I was becoming a one-man EMS publicity department. FDNY administrators, meanwhile, were putting all their energy into making firefighters look good. They lined up fire trucks outside emergency departments to cheer health workers. They were following the lead of ordinary New Yorkers, who had started to applaud and bang pots every night to thank first responders. New Yorkers were doing other things too, like putting up handwritten thank-you signs and rainbows in windows and offering free coffee to first responders at diners. It was touching and it lifted our spirits—everybody's spirits, I think.

The FDNY clapping went over very well with the public. What people didn't realize was that the reason New York's Bravest had time to clap for health workers was that they had been instructed not to respond to COVID calls. They were sitting on the sidelines while we ran into people's houses.

Mike and I hadn't seen each other since the pandemic hit. We hadn't had any time, and we worked and lived at opposite ends of the city. But we'd been checking in with each other every day. We always do. A text, a call. Angie does that too if we don't cross paths at work. Other people check on their parents or their kids or whoever they care about most. That's what we were doing.

I had come straight from work. "Man, you look worn out," Mike said.

He set up the light and the tripod. I recorded an interview with Ali Velshi from MSNBC. I hadn't yet mastered the art of looking straight at the interviewer. I was distracted by my own image on the screen and my eyes kept darting to the left. But I said what I need to say.

Velshi brought up the EMS pay issue. I talked about attrition.

"You want twenty-year people," I said. "To be training new people and to be treating you and your families. Unfortunately, with the way this city is treating EMS, that's not the case."

After the Velshi interview, I was invited to go to the CNN studio and talk to Poppy Harlow. A morning news show! This was big.

For the interview, I wore a dark gray EMS jacket and a light blue EMS shirt. I had worked a double shift the day before. I had hardly slept. I looked like I'd been hit by a truck. But that was authentic. No point looking healthy and well rested when you're representing a group of people who are on their knees. I described the call to Sheepshead Bay, how I couldn't comfort the guy who lost his wife. My voice cracked. How was that man? I wondered. Had he made it? Was he watching?

Help came from unexpected places. One day in the middle of the mayhem, three men knocked on the door of the station. They ran a pharmacy in Sunset Park, and they had made hand sanitizer. They brought boxes of it, piled on the sidewalk. They wanted to donate it to us. We led the guys into the apparatus floor. They were from Chennai in southern India. We talked about India. We huddled together for a photo.

The men from Chennai weren't the only ones who helped out. Pornhub, the internet porn site, donated fifteen thousand masks to EMS and thousands more to other first responders in the New York area. I have no idea why Pornhub decided to help us. Probably good publicity. After all, who knew better than Pornhub the importance of personal protection? But the fire department wasn't amused, and I could understand why. It said a lot about the fire department's incompetence that an internet pornography company had to bail us out.

Toward the end of March, Station 40 had a bit of karma. Karma on a motorbike.

My phone rang. It was Jose Rosario. "Anthony, I'd like to come and feed the station houses," Jose said.

Jose was the president of a motorcycle club, the Hustle Kingz. He was a big, round guy with a goatee. He'd grown up in the industrial section of Sunset Park. The bikers were mainly city employees. They did ride-outs for breast cancer, autism. They could distribute food, he said.

Jose was dating Sol-Luz, who'd gone to my elementary school. In June 2019, I bumped into Sol and Jose in the emergency department at Lutheran Hospital. It was around the time of Joe's retirement party. Jose had skidded on wet leaves and crashed his Kawasaki. He was banged up, but not too seriously. I walked Jose over to one of the emergency department nurses, told her that he was a friend, and asked her to take care of him. After that, we stayed in touch.

"There's a lot of restaurants that are closed," Jose said over the phone. "They need people to cook for. And you guys are going through the most difficult time in your history."

True. The crews were eating every meal in the ambulance or at the station. Many of the local restaurants were closed. Nobody had time to cook. Nobody had time to shop, especially not when lines at stores were going around the block. Plus, some EMTs felt uncomfortable going into stores in uniform. They felt that the store owners feared they were contaminated.

"Do you really think you can pull this off?" I asked Jose.

"Watch me," he said.

A few days later, very early, Jose arrived at Station 40 with a big spread: Bagels, butter, cream cheese. Croissants. Orange juice, coffee. His bikers had pooled their money and reached out to a local spot called Sunset Bagels. And here they were, with a breakfast fit for a king. Or a hungry EMS worker.

After that, Jose organized meals for other stations. A motorcycle stunt rider with restaurant connections hooked him up with cooks around the city. Jose asked for donations from his friends, from bikers, from people he'd known when he worked security for rap artists, from Instagram connections. Whoever he could reach.

A seafood restaurant in Queens delivered food to EMS stations there. A keto chef in East New York cooked for the stations nearby. A former workmate of Jose made oxtail stew. For a month, give or take, Jose took food to EMS stations in every borough, all of it delivered by men and women on huge, shiny motorbikes. The Brooklyn cavalry had arrived.

Also unexpectedly, I received a text message from my sister, Yvonne.

Yvonne and I hadn't spoken for a few years. We'd stayed in touch after my parents died, seen each other occasionally—but then we had an argument about money. Yvonne had wanted her daughter Amanda to take out a mortgage for a property in New Jersey that Yvonne planned to turn into a pizzeria (Yvonne had moved to New Jersey in 2013). I'd advised Amanda against it. Amanda was a bright bulb, but in my opinion, Yvonne leaned on her too much. The last thing Amanda needed was to potentially be saddled with Yvonne's debt.

I felt a responsibility toward my nieces and nephews. Not because we were close but because I'd extracted myself from the family dysfunction and I hated to see them still caught up in it. Especially Anthony, Richie's son. I felt like I should've taken him with me when I left. I told him that a few years ago. Anthony had grown up with his mother, Holly, and her mom and my mom. He didn't finish high school. He'd never had a steady job that I knew of. He lived in Staten Island and occasionally hung out with a rough crowd. It was too late for me to help him turn things around.

Amanda, though, I figured I could do something for. But Yvonne had been very offended. So we'd lost touch. She'd gone on to open the pizzeria with Amanda's help, an arrangement that turned out much like I'd feared it would.

Yvonne texted me from time to time, but I didn't always respond. I just didn't have the energy to argue with her. This time, though, was different. Yvonne was checking to see if I was okay.

I was wiping down the command car at the start of my shift when my phone buzzed.

Hey, Anthony. I saw you on TV. How you holding up?

I put down the cleaning supplies, wiped my hands. Okay, I wrote. How about u?

Okay. Everything shut down. Pizza is takeout only.

At least the pizza business is still alive, I thought.

I was surprised by how good it felt to hear from Yvonne. I had stopped relying on her emotionally a long time ago. In fact, one of the reasons I avoided contact was that I found her exhausting. She always wanted to talk about her childhood, about our parents. Every story involved her being a hard-ass and getting her own way. She shared that with my mother—they both felt that the world was against them and that they had to get even with people.

But I was touched that she'd thought of me.

Glad the pizza place is okay, I wrote. Then: Don't play around with this virus. Mask up. Wash your hands.

We do. You think it'll get worse?

Yep, I wrote. Gotta go. Work is crazy. Then I added, Thanks for the message.

Stay safe, Anthony, she wrote. I'm proud of you.

APRIL 2020

S unday morning. Cropsey Avenue. Cardiac arrest.

I pulled up outside the nursing home as Stephen Northmore and his partner parked their ambulance ahead of me. A fire truck was already at the scene. Northmore and his partner climbed out. Pulled on gowns. Then a second pair of gloves.

Northmore was a guy who took things seriously—the pandemic being a case in point—and he was meticulous with PPE. That's part of what separates a very experienced medic from a rookie. Northmore changed his gloves constantly. He put a pair of gloves on over his first pair before he treated a patient, then took them off before he wheeled or carried the patient out of the apartment. That way, he avoided touching a COVID patient and then contaminating the doorknob of an apartment building that multiple people touched every hour. Northmore often changed his gloves again when he got back to the ambulance, since there was no point in sanitizing your ambulance if you were going to contaminate it with whatever you had just picked up from the door handle.

As Northmore would say, you don't think about how many things you touch during a call until you get feces on your gloves. Then you realize that you touch just about everything: The patient, the blood pressure cuff, the stair chair, your medical bag, your mask. The patient-care report tablet, the doorknob, the elevator button, the keys to the ambulance. The stretcher, the bench, the captain's chair, the monitor, the cabinets where we stow equipment, the on-board oxygen gauge, the radio mike.

We all piled into an elevator—a pair of firefighters, Northmore, his partner, me. No social distancing here. We leaned against the elevator walls. Weary.

"Another arrest," I said.

"You caught any yet today, Lou?"

"This is my fourth."

It was 8:27 a.m.

That morning, I had logged on to the truck at just after six. It was April 5. The pandemic was in full swing. The day before, the number of cases of COVID-19 registered in the city had hit 60,850. Governor Cuomo, who held daily briefings on the battle with the virus, said that 594 people in the state had died of the virus that day. Nearly all of them were in New York City. Emergency Dispatch was receiving more than six thousand calls a day. EMTs and paramedics often worked back-to-back tours, sixteen hours. Then they stripped off their uniforms, put them in a red bag, drove home, showered, ate, slept, woke up, and returned to work.

The crush was so bad that the Federal Emergency Management Agency had sent two hundred fifty ambulances and EMT crews to New York to help. The crews were picking up the less urgent jobs, feeling their way around an alien city gripped by a plague. The U.S. military had turned the Javits Center, a convention center in Manhattan, into a temporary hospital. A gigantic white military hospital ship, the USNS *Mercy*, had docked in the Hudson. FEMA also sent dozens of additional medical examiners and refrigerated trucks. Even so, we could barely keep pace with the dead.

I was beat before I'd even arrived at work that morning. Everyone was exhausted. We'd been in a tunnel for two weeks, and we didn't know where it ended. The only thing we knew was that we'd never catch up. All these calls; all these people waiting. I had worked hurricanes and heat waves. During Hurricane Sandy, we had crews carrying patients down ten flights of stairs in buildings with no power. It was chaos. But it lasted two days and then it was over—for EMS, at least.

This was different. The pandemic felt endless, like going fifteen rounds with Mike Tyson when Tyson was in his prime, then fifteen more. And there was nowhere to hide. You hit the button to go available after you transferred a patient and—boom!—you were hit with a job. You took a break to run to the bathroom and—boom!—you were hit with a job.

When I arrived at the station that Sunday morning, the lieutenant from the night tour was finishing up. She put the radio and the keys to the command vehicle on the table outside the lieutenants' office. We didn't pass things hand to hand if we could avoid it. I took a disinfectant wipe. I had a box of Clorox wipes that had been in my house for months that I'd barely used, but now I was rationing them, using a couple to clean my equipment on each new tour.

I asked if the call volume had been high overnight. Crazy, the lieutenant said, till about three, when it calmed down. Crazy-busy wasn't unusual for Saturday nights; they were always busier than other nights. People got drunk, got high, got into fights, crashed their cars. But now, with everybody shut up at home, that kind of thing wasn't why we were getting so many calls. It was the virus.

After a short lull—people sleeping, most likely—the radio had started ticking again, the lieutenant said. And the truck needed gas.

I ran out to fill up the gas tank and get myself a bagel. The spots where I usually got breakfast were closed, so I drove thirty blocks to La Bagel Delight, the store in Park Slope where I'd worked when I was just out of high school. The store had moved a couple of blocks down Seventh Avenue since my day, but some of the old crew was still there. I ordered a toasted everything with a schmear of scallion cream cheese, lox, and sliced red onion. I got a Martinelli's apple juice. The cashier had hung a clear plastic garbage bag in front of the register to protect himself. I ate the bagel in the truck.

The first call came in just before six thirty: cardiac arrest, elderly man, nursing home south of Prospect Park.

The streets were deserted, so I got to the scene quickly. The nursing home was an awful place. It was grubby and smelled of urine, and the staff acted like they couldn't care less about the patients. I'd been there many times. It was one of the first homes to have a big COVID outbreak.

When I reached the patient's room, he was dead. Suspected COVID. I checked in with the crews there, handed them a few bottles of water. *Everyone okay?* I asked. *Remember to keep hydrated.*

I went back out, wiped down the truck again, and hit the button. "Conditions Four-O."

The next assignment was another cardiac arrest—no surprise—two miles south in Bay Ridge. A man lay in a bedroom of a small brick house, unresponsive. His family said that he had had a fever and cough for a few days. We started CPR. The medics intubated him so that they could breathe for him. We performed CPR for about half an hour, rotating providers every two minutes. No pulse. No breathing. We pronounced the man dead.

Next stop, a Chinese guy in an apartment building in Borough Park. His grandson had come to visit him and found him in bed, unconscious. We couldn't revive him.

Another cardiac arrest. My third of the morning.

COVID-19 wrecks the body in multiple ways. It starves the tissues of oxygen. The organs, including the heart, begin to fail. The heart stops pumping blood properly. The patient goes into cardiac arrest. Biological death occurs within six minutes, give or take.

In April 2020, the number of cardiac arrests in New York City went through the roof. Emergency medical dispatchers normally log 80 or so cardiac arrests in the city each day. In early April, they were logging an average of 300. The number peaked at 407. Not many of those patients survived.

One reason for this was that people were waiting too long before they called 911. They were afraid to go to the hospital. They had heard about people lying in corridors and dying alone in the ICU, so they stuck it out at home until they were so sick that their lungs or their hearts gave out.

And the official tally doesn't tell the whole story. A lot of calls that came over the system as a fever/cough or a diff breather ended up with the patient in cardiac arrest. These patients had been conscious when they or their relatives called. But their hearts had stopped working by the time we arrived. That's not unheard of, but now it was happening time after time.

This surge in cardiac arrests put huge demand on resources, especially paramedics. Of all the hands we send to an arrest—an EMT unit, a paramedic unit, and a fire truck—paramedics are the most important. Only they can provide advanced life support.

But FDNY paramedics are scarce at the best of times; my station has only one paramedic unit, the ambulance that Angie and Jimmy work on. And with so many members of FDNY EMS on medical leave—at the end of the first week of April, one in four was out—paramedics were as rare as unicorns.

So EMTs were thrown into the deep end. It was awful to listen to desperate dispatchers sending EMT crews unaided to calls that would normally require a paramedic unit. "ALS extended," they would say, indicating that the nearest paramedics were far away, or "No ALS available."

"Conditions Four-O for the assignment. Back up Four-Two Boy for the cardiac arrest. No ALS available."

"Four-Two Adam, Seventy-First Street and Fourteenth Avenue for the fever/cough. No ALS available. No conditions car available."

"Six-Five John take it over to Fourth Avenue and Thirty-Eighth Street for the arrest fever/cough. No ALS available."

"Four-Three George for Fort Hamilton and Fifty-Eighth Street. Fever/cough. ALS extended. Coming from Brooklyn Central."

On and on it went, hour after hour: No ALS. No ALS.

Don't get sick, New Yorkers, I thought. *Because there's nobody here to save you.*

Ten minutes after I left the Chinese patient in Borough Park that Sunday, I took the call at the nursing home on Cropsey, which was where I ran into Stephen Northmore.

Cropsey Avenue runs parallel to the sea, from Bensonhurst to Coney Island, Italy to Russia. It's lined with nursing homes. I guess the idea was that the elderly folks who lived there would get some sea air. In reality, they never leave the facilities. And now those facilities had become hotbeds of COVID.

We would learn only later just how many people died in nursing homes in New York State. So many that Governor Cuomo's office disguised the death toll until an investigation by the attorney general's office in January 2021 revealed the true scope of the losses. An analysis by the *New York Times* put the number of nursing-home residents who died of the virus through June 2021 at nearly sixteen thousand. Most of those people died during the fateful spring of 2020.

Seeing these old people dying alone made me mad. What were they doing here? I wondered as I rode up on the elevator with Northmore, his partner, and the two firefighters. When the pandemic was coming, why did families leave them here? Why didn't they get them out? Take them home? People must have known that the nursing homes would be incubators for the virus.

The elevator doors opened, and Northmore and his partner and I headed down the corridor to the patient's room while the firefighters waited behind. The patient was on the bed, very frail. She was ninety years old. A doctor and a nurse were performing chest compressions, but the patient looked dead. Stiff jaw. Pale, dry skin. They were trying to revive a corpse. If she didn't have a DNR, they had a legal obligation to try.

"When did she lose consciousness?" Northmore asked.

The nurse looked up. "I'm going to be honest," she said. "Nobody is sure when this patient was last seen alive."

The nurse was from out of town. Thousands of nurses from other parts of the country had come to New York to relieve nurses who had fallen sick. The nurses from out of town thought many of the nursing homes in New York were terrible places. Which they were.

The nurse shrugged. "I don't even know if you want to work this patient up," she said. She lifted the patient gently to reveal her back. The skin was purplish. This is what's known as dependent lividity, and it occurs when blood pools in the lowest part of the deceased person's body, a process that usually begins about half an hour after death. The patient was long gone.

Northmore turned to me. His look said: *What do you think?*

"She's right," I said. "I'll call telemetry. We'll pronounce her."

Less than an hour later, I was standing in a green park near the sea, examining another corpse. A young corpse this time. And not a COVID patient. And this one, at least, had died in the open air, with the smell of the sea blowing off the strait between Brooklyn and Staten Island.

The man had chosen an odd way to kill himself. The tree was not particularly tall. It was shaped like a Christmas tree. The man lay underneath the tree, his feet and legs trailing on the grass. His neck was tied to a branch with the cord of a phone charger. The branch was only a foot or so clear of the grass, so the man's body sloped toward the ground like a person doing a push-up or a plank.

Someone out for an early walk had called the cops. The neighborhood, at the southern tip of Bay Ridge, was very suburban. Opposite the park were brick row houses and a Catholic school. Beyond those was the blue of the sea.

The guy wore a dark-colored hoodie. He looked to be in his late twenties. On the grass next to the tree was a book bag and a liquor bottle. Apparently, he'd tied the cord of a phone charger around the branch, looped it around his neck, then relaxed his arms and legs and let the cord do its work. That was not a peaceful way to die. Or an efficient one. Some suicides climb onto a chair and kick it away. If things go as planned, their neck breaks when they drop. The way this man killed himself, there was no drop. His neck didn't break. He just hung with the cord digging into his throat until he suffocated. He must have felt everything.

Two cops stood by, along with an EMT crew from my house, Station 40. One of the EMTs was Arnold Chen, the one who'd sworn he'd never catch COVID.

I held my fingers to the guy's carotid. No pulse. His body was cold and stiff. "He's dead for sure," I said. Then: "At least he doesn't have COVID."

I was relieved. The guy had killed himself in a bizarre way, but he had ended his life by choice. If there was anything to explain, it wasn't my job to do it. But all the deaths of the past few weeks? The people with COVID? The people who weren't too sick one day and were dead the next? We didn't know how to explain those.

The cops would stay with the body. We had nothing more to do here. I chatted for a moment with the EMTs. How were they doing? A lot of cardiac arrests? Had they transported anyone?

"It's crazy," Chen said. That's what we all said every day: *It's crazy out there.*

After the update, Chen and his partner walked back to their ambulance. I pulled down my mask and breathed through my nose. I could smell the salt water. I took a long breath. I would have been content to stand next to this corpse for a while just to get a few minutes of quiet.

At the next call, I think we broke a woman's heart. The neighborhood wasn't far from the station. Limestone houses with bay windows, tall stoops. I headed inside with a medic crew from a private hospital. I knew one of the medics, Mariana, a tough woman with a prominent jaw.

A woman was kneeling on the floor of the living room, bent over the body of her mother, pushing on her chest. She was not pushing nearly hard enough—people without training rarely do. The medics jumped in and took over. The younger woman stood up. I took her into the bedroom, and she explained that her mother had been sick for few days with COVID symptoms. Suddenly, she'd stopped breathing.

"You were here on Thursday," the woman added. "For my father. He had the symptoms too. He didn't make it."

I ducked back into the living room. *Shit.* This woman's dad had just died of COVID, and I wanted to be able to tell the woman, *We got your mom back!* But when Mariana looked up, her eyes told me all I needed to know. There was no life in this body. No hope of reviving her. I would have to tell the woman that she had now lost both parents. Three days apart.

Afterward, I stood outside with the medic crew. I wondered when the woman would be able to hold funerals for her parents. The funeral parlors were so backed up, she might wait months, and then one day, she would have to say goodbye to both of them at once.

I thought that life had trained me for the pandemic. I'd experienced a lot of death: my brother, Richie; some other family members; some friends. And I'd seen a lot during my nearly two decades working 911 in New York.

I got this, I'd thought. *Death is my wheelhouse.*

But the pandemic was like nothing else. It feasted on New York. At the end of the first week of April, New York City recorded more than eight hundred COVID-related deaths in a single day. For a week after that, a New Yorker died every two minutes. They died in intensive care units. On COVID wards. At home. On the sidewalk. In the backs of ambulances.

At first, adrenaline got me through. It was like surfing and crashing on a big wave. You go under and then you pop up. But after a few days, as the waves kept coming, it became harder and harder to get above the water.

As a lieutenant, I'm the one who pronounces the time of death if it occurs on a call. I'm the one who offers condolences to the family, who tells them what we did to try to save the person and why we weren't able to do it. The scenes can be incredibly emotional: The explosion of disbelief. The screams that fill the room.

Because I've been doing this for years, though, I am calm in these situations. I sit with the family for a few minutes. I put an arm around a shoulder. I try to share a little in their grief. It's a responsibility to bear witness to people's loss, and I consider it a privilege. But in the spring of 2020, I went from one house to the next telling families that their father or uncle or mother or grandmother or husband or son or daughter was gone.

And when you pronounce four people dead before lunch, the well of empathy, of perspective—it starts to run dry.

That Sunday became a blur. House, apartment, nursing home. Bay Ridge, Bath Beach, Sunset Park. Grandpa, uncle, mother, son. I responded to fourteen calls in sixteen hours. I traced a miserable zigzag across Brooklyn. Almost every patient presented with symptoms of COVID.

Every patient died.

There was a thirty-five-year-old man who collapsed on the sidewalk as his roommate tried to walk him to the nearest emergency room. There was the father of a doctor in a 1930s building south of Prospect Park. *Even with all my knowledge, I couldn't save him,* the daughter said.

Late lunchtime, I went back to the station to use the bathroom. I picked up some more masks, offered to fetch something to eat for Stan Flaksman, the lieutenant sitting the desk that day. He said he was good. Stan lived on granola bars and protein shakes.

I opened the back door of the truck and sat with my legs dangling. I stared at my hands. I was shattered. It's hubris to think we can always save people, that we can give them life. It's egotistical. I recognize that. But on the job, it's what sustains you, that possibility you can save someone. And we weren't saving anybody.

"You okay, Anthony?"

It was Northmore, the medic who had been with me at the nursing home.

"I dunno," I said. "There's a lot of death out there."

"You're telling me," Northmore said. A couple of hours after I'd seen him at the nursing home, he'd gone to another home on Cropsey Avenue for an elderly patient who was in respiratory failure. He and his partner had transported the patient to a hospital near the ocean. When they'd arrived there, a medic who was on his way out of the emergency department had warned them that it was mayhem inside, that there were several patients in respiratory failure and only two doctors.

"We walked in and the look on the doctor's face—it was panic," Northmore said. "He and this other doctor were bouncing between the patients. He was shouting at us, 'You've gotta stop bringing them here. You've gotta take them somewhere else!'"

Northmore said he wanted to take my picture because he liked the light. It was very clear, he said. Probably because there was less pollution than normal. Angie walked over with Alex Tepily. They were working together that day. They were about to start their tour.

"How's it going out there, Anthony?" Angie asked.

"It's hell," I said.

We decided to take a group photo. We set a timer on Flaksman's phone and propped it on a stretcher. Antonio Ruvolo, a new EMT, joined the group and stood the farthest to my left. Opposite him, Flaksman wore a mask. He said his wife would freak if she saw him without one. Tepily stood next to Flaksman. Angie managed a smile. Not her wide, white-teeth smile; just a regular smile. I look grim. I have a furrow between my brows. The sides of my mouth tip downward. Next to me, Northmore also looks serious. But he was right about the light—it was kind of nice. Like the light that you get on a mountain.

• • •

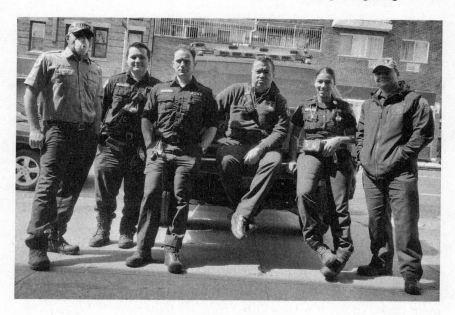

Cardiac arrest number twelve. Late afternoon. I pushed open the front door to a two-story brick house with a red awning in Bay Ridge. We ask patients to leave the door open when they call. Too often, a patient calls and then collapses unconscious and we have to force entry.

I followed the sound of voices through the living room and into the kitchen. It was very tidy. A family stood there in a huddle. I believe they were Chinese. Next door, there was a bedroom. A pair of EMTs and a pair of medics knelt beside a man in his fifties, also Chinese. The medics looked up when they heard me enter. I knew one of them: Mariana. We kept crossing paths that day.

The medics' eyes were dead. Usually, when we work on a patient, there's a lot of adrenaline; we're really focused on bringing the patient back, even though we know the odds are often small. There's an energy to it. But these medics had a flat stare. I swear that the patient had more life in his eyes.

I turned to the family. They were all wearing masks. Very quiet. I told them that I was there to help the crew. One of the family members was a kid, eighteen or nineteen years old. He appeared to be the only person who spoke English. He talked to a middle-aged woman in what I assume was Mandarin.

"What's going on?" the teenager asked me. The man on the floor was his uncle, he said. The woman was his mother.

"Your uncle is very sick," I said. "The crew is seeing what they can do. He has no pulse. He's not breathing. We are breathing for him. We're doing CPR. They are going to start an IV on him and give him medication to see if we can get his heart to beat again. He's getting the same medication that he'd get in a hospital."

We were giving him epinephrine, sodium bicarbonate, and dextrose in the IV. Epinephrine constricts the blood vessels and increases coronary perfusion (the blood supply to the heart muscle). Sodium bicarbonate helps balance acids in the blood. Dextrose boosts blood sugar.

The teenager translated. His mother made little nodding movements as he spoke. Her eyes flitted from me to her son. We often come across younger family members who translate for parents and grandparents. They act as translators for everything—school meetings, doctor's appointments. It's a lot of responsibility.

For twenty minutes or so, the crews worked on the patient. The guy had been short of breath for a few days, the teenager said. As I looked at the family, I couldn't help wondering if any of them were infected. They were clearly being careful—masking up, keeping their distance from us—but if they were all living under this one roof, infection was almost inevitable.

The patient was in asystole, meaning his heart emitted no electrical impulses. It did not pump or flutter. On the cardiac monitor, it presented as a flat line.

So now I had to give the speech. I had it down. I could have delivered it in my sleep.

I pulled the teenager aside. "I need you to translate what I am going to say," I told him. "Your uncle—we intubated him. We started an IV. We did CPR for more than twenty minutes. We gave him all the medications that we could. He still has no pulse."

The kid looked at me as if to say, *So?*

"I'm very sorry. There's nothing more that we can do."

The kid's mother said something. She sounded desperate. He snapped at her. Then he turned back to me. He was agitated.

"No," he said. "You have to go back in there. You have to wake him up."

Most of his face was covered by his mask. I could only see his eyes, darting back and forth.

"He can't be dead," he said. "You have to take him to the hospital. You have to do more."

It was understandable. Patients' families want to believe that something more can be done, that the outcome will change if the patient goes to the hospital. In normal times, we might have loaded the man and transported him, even if it was just to comfort the family.

But the medical system was so swamped during the pandemic that our protocols had changed. As of March 31, we were transporting patients only if we got a pulse back at the scene. Hospitals didn't have the resources to try to resuscitate them, and we didn't have the resources to transport them, so we had to pronounce these patients dead then and there.

We'd also been told not to transport patients with COVID-like symptoms to the hospital unless they had underlying medical conditions or were over sixty-five—unless they were high risk, in other words. Other patients were given a hotline number and an information sheet about how to deal with symptoms and contain the spread of the disease. Those patients were on their own.

I looked the kid in the eye. "We can't get a pulse," I said again. "There's nothing we can do. Can you please explain to your mother?"

The kid tensed. His body shifted. He squared his shoulders. He looked like he was about to take a swing at me. I felt my pulse quicken. I took a step back.

The mother said something in Mandarin. The kid started to pace. I pulled my mask down. I wanted him to see me as a person.

"I need you to look at me," I said. I wasn't shouting, but I raised my voice. "There's nothing we can do. We can't bring him back."

The kid's eyes settled on my face.

"You need to be here for your mom," I said. "There will be time to be angry. But right now, she needs you."

I pulled up my mask. The kid went over and stood with his mother. He put his arm around her shoulder. In the other room, the medics were packing up. I told the kid that one of the EMTs would stay with his uncle until the cops came to take his body to the morgue.

We left the house, and I sat down on the stoop. My eyes stung. My breath came quickly. I was boiling with rage for the kid, for the city, for me. The kind of anger you feel as a child when things are out of your control. When everything has gone wrong and there's nothing you can do to change it.

Why the fuck am I here? I thought. *Why is this kid's uncle dead?* He'd probably come to the United States with his sister to build a new life. And he had lost that life for no reason.

People like him were dying because they had to go to work. Or because they couldn't go and hide in the Hamptons. Or because they'd lost their jobs and, with them, their health insurance. And the government hadn't shut down soon enough. The kid was right to be upset. And I was an asshole for telling him to calm down.

"Lou, are you okay?"

It was Mariana. She sat down next to me on the stoop.

"I don't know what I'm doing anymore," I said, choking up.

Mariana said nothing. She put her arm around me. We sat in silence for a minute or so. Then I slowly got to my feet.

"Thanks," I said. "Let's go get the next one."

A little after nine o'clock that night, I started heading back to the station, dizzy with fatigue. Since breakfast, I'd done eleven cardiac arrests and the suicide. Twelve calls, twelve deaths. I hadn't eaten since the bagel; I'd just chugged Red Bull all day. I needed to sit down and put something in my stomach. But it wasn't meant to be.

"Conditions Four-O for the arrest on Fifth Avenue and Thirty-Sixth Street. Back up Four-Two Boy."

Four-Two Boy was Bones's unit. At least I'd be on this call with him. I did a U-turn and headed north.

I stopped my truck outside a small apartment building opposite Green-Wood Cemetery, a beautiful area on a hill just north of Sunset Park. During lockdown, people started taking walks along the paths between the graves and crypts. But it was night, and the gates would be locked. Nobody would be walking there now except the ghosts.

Bones and his partner pulled up in their ambulance. "Major injury?" said Bones.

"No, it's an arrest," I said.

"Jeez. ALS?"

"They'll be a while. They're extended. Coming from Brooklyn Central."

We needed a paramedic crew in case we had to intubate the patient and to help with CPR. But the nearest paramedic crew was twenty minutes away, and one of the members of that crew normally had a desk job, coordinating Brooklyn's paramedic teams. We were stretched so thin that he was working on the road. We'd have to manage without them for now. I could help out with CPR. My injured arm made it hard for me to lift things, but with my arms locked straight, I could pump a chest for two minutes.

The house across from Green-Wood was occupied by a Spanish-speaking family. Mexican, I believe. The apartment was cluttered. There were crucifixes and pictures of Christ on the walls of the living room. There was a bed of some kind in the room, and the patient was on the bed. Bones and his partner lowered him to the floor; the family helped. He was eighty-two years old. Bald. His skin was ocher-colored. Bones felt for a pulse and then started chest compressions. His partner bagged the patient (pushed air into his lungs through a bag-mask device). I spoke to the family and then took over pumping the man's chest. There were only three of us.

As we worked, the family stood around us in a circle. I heard them muttering in Spanish. I couldn't understand what they said, but when I looked up, I saw that they had stretched their arms above our heads in the shape of a tepee. As we knelt beneath them, compressing the grandfather's chest, they chanted in prayer.

But God didn't answer.

When we got back to the station, Bones peeled off his uniform, put everything into a bag to take home and wash, then went into the restroom to clean up. The door was propped open. I sat on a chair and watched him as he washed his hands, then took a paper towel and balled it up and ran it around the inside of his nose. Next, he scrubbed his face with his fingertips. Little motions, around and around. It was like he was lost in time. Scrub, scrub. Like he was trying to get the death off his skin.

April 5 was my day from hell, the worst one in terms of the number of deaths I witnessed. Seven hundred and fifty people died of COVID-19 in New York City that day according to the official tally. But every day in early April was much the same for EMS and hospital workers in New York City. Units tore from one cardiac arrest to the next. Every EMS station in the city was understaffed. It was like being in a hurricane when you can hear nothing except the howl of the wind.

"We have our foot to the floor, and the engine is at redline," Governor Cuomo said during a press briefing on April 6. Hospitals couldn't sustain the pace for any amount of time, he said, "because the system will blow."

At the end of the first week of April, I saw a post on Facebook from Johana Clerge, my friend at Station 59. I hadn't spoken to Johana since the city locked down, but we'd texted a few times. We were both run ragged.

I don't know where to begin, Johana wrote on Facebook. The post was a few days old. *I know I will never be the same mentally because of my work.*

On April 2, Johana had worked a sixteen-hour day. She'd pronounced fourteen patients dead. Johana had four kids in school. At the time, they were all in remote learning, so after a day on the road, Johana went home, fixed them food, and helped them navigate online classes.

Johana's mother lived near her in Canarsie and April 2 was her birthday. Between cardiac arrests, Johana had rushed to a bakery and bought a cake, then driven to her mother's home. There was a chair in the garden that people would sit on while Johana's mother stood on her balcony. Johana had put the cake on the chair and waved to her mother. Then she'd gone to another cardiac arrest.

In my 16 years of being in FDNY EMS I never had a day like I had yesterday, Johana wrote. *I watched some of my crews break down. I cried on the phone,* she went on. *I even had a panic attack in my vehicle.*

The day she posted that message on Facebook, Johana asked her fellow lieutenant if it would be okay if she sat the desk at the station from then on. For the first time in her career, she didn't want to be on the road. She couldn't take it anymore.

And then the storm died down. The swell of sickness that had washed over New York City subsided almost as quickly as it had risen. On April 12, the volume of medical calls to 911 dipped below five thousand for the first time in weeks. Fewer people were being hospitalized—in the middle of the month, it was about a thousand a day; on April 1, the daily average had been about sixteen hundred. The number of people dying in New York City had also begun to fall, from a high of over eight hundred a day at the end of the first week in April to below five hundred on April 21. By the end of April, EMS was fielding under four thousand calls per day, close to our regular call volume. Deaths had fallen to below three hundred daily, and the average number of people being admitted to the hospital was around three hundred a day.

There were probably a few reasons for the drop in calls. The fire department had gotten the message across that you shouldn't call 911 unless it was a true emergency. People also had been shut indoors for a month, so the virus was spreading less quickly. And they were finally wearing masks, even outdoors. Andrew Cuomo made masks mandatory in mid-April. A little late, but still.

Plus, a lot of people had died. It was that simple. The city said at the time that between March 11 and April 13, COVID-19 had claimed 10,367 lives. The true toll was probably thousands more. But in any case, there were a lot of New Yorkers who simply were no longer around to call 911.

We knew that the virus hadn't gone away. We dreaded another wave like the one that had just hit us. But the lull gave us a moment to catch our breath.

Mercifully, we had also had gotten help carrying some of the load.

The FEMA ambulances and crews that had come from other parts of the country were spread around New York. Most people were stationed near an EMS station or a police precinct. They slept at hotels or in dormitories at Fort Totten, a former army installation in Queens where the FDNY EMS Academy is located. During the day, FEMA crews sat on their intersections and picked up lower-priority calls, taking some of the heat off New York–based ambulance crews. It was a help, and it was nice to have EMS members from out of town. They were making good money, but that didn't change the fact that they'd volunteered to come to the heart of the pandemic, to a city they had no connection to. It took guts. Bones, especially, loved it. No more old people who couldn't get off the toilet. No more cut fingers. The FEMA ambulances were picking up those calls.

• • •

Our reprieve didn't last long. Because just as the surge in 911 calls started dropping, we began to lose colleagues to the virus.

One of them was Tony Thomas, my instructor in paramedic school. Tony, who was always putting off retirement. Tony, who was always "almost there" but holding on for that extra financial security. Tony had been working on a hospital ambulance in March when he caught COVID. He died on April 12.

That month, the fire department lost at least ten members to COVID. Four were emergency medical workers: John Redd, a sixty-three-year-old emergency medical dispatcher who had been with the service for twenty-six years and was working in the Dispatch office during the crisis; Idris Bey, a twenty-seven-year veteran of the department who was a certified first responder instructor at Fort Totten; and Richard Seaberry, an EMT in Queens who had been in EMS for thirty years. The fourth EMS fatality was Greg Hodge, my mentor from the early days in Harlem—the former Delta pilot with the beautiful, lilting voice. Greg died on April 12, the same day as Tony.

He had remained an EMT for all those years. He'd worked in Harlem and then the Bronx. He had been part of the rescue and recovery effort on September 11, 2001. And then he'd gone to work at the New York City Office of Emergency Management, which plans and coordinates disaster response. There, Greg had been watch commander, a role that had him working with first responders in the field and keeping tabs on everything that went on during an emergency through radio frequencies, news channels, weather reports, and the emergency dispatch system.

In March 2020, Greg had been tasked with taking workers' temperatures and had had contact with a worker who was infected.

Greg was sick for about ten days. He developed a fever. The fever came and went—a few days of fever, a day without. Greg isolated himself in his apartment, and his fiancée, Nancy, checked on him by phone. Greg was a keen tennis player and a cyclist and he had powerful lungs. But about nine days into the illness, he started to cough, Nancy said.

That day, Greg told Nancy that his pet bird was going crazy. Flying all over the apartment. It was a bird of paradise. Greg had had the bird for years. He told Nancy he was going to put the bird back in its cage and go rest, and he'd text her when he woke up. The next morning, Nancy still hadn't heard from Greg. She called him, but he didn't answer. A few more hours passed and Nancy began to worry. She called Greg's office to alert them and headed to his apartment.

When Nancy arrived, there were two ambulances, a car from Emergency Management, and fire trucks parked outside his building. She peeked into the backs of the ambulances. She knew that once Greg was in the hospital, there would be no way to visit him. She wanted to see him before he was transported. But the ambulances were empty.

Nick Magro, a Harlem paramedic who worked with Greg, came out of the building. He broke the news to Nancy. He started to cry.

Nancy wasn't allowed to go inside. The risk of infection was too high. David Deleon, a lieutenant paramedic from Greg's former station in Harlem, kept watch over Greg until the medical examiner came. David sat in the room for hours. Greg looked like he was sleeping, he told Nancy. His bird escaped from the cage and hid under the bed. When the medical examiner came to take Greg's body, the bird flew up and flapped around the room. It didn't want to let them move him.

Although we were getting help from the out-of-town crews, we still weren't getting support from our chiefs. Apparently, they were working from home. And when we did get a message from on high, it was in the form of a memo about yet another change in protocol.

Our protocols were shifting constantly. What protective equipment to wear, how to deal with a cardiac arrest, whether to consult telemetry about where to take a patient, whether to consult telemetry before pronouncing a patient, whether to notify the hospital if you were transporting a suspected case of COVID, how often to change your N95 mask.

It was bewildering and annoying. And it was an unnecessary source of anxiety in the middle of a major shitshow. In a job where you have to make life-and-death decisions on the fly, clear protocols are crucial. They give you a framework to operate in. New rules take time to adjust to, and they were being thrown at us every day.

On April 17, the city's department of health published new standards for prehospital resuscitation. If we didn't get a pulse back or detect electrical activity in the heart—in other words, if the patient was in asystole—we should stop CPR after twenty minutes and pronounce the patient dead.

That was a significant change. New York City emergency medical workers don't have a time limit on CPR. We can work on a patient until we're convinced there's no chance of resuscitation. We can keep up CPR all the way to the hospital, where the emergency department has tools to stabilize a patient. They can start a central line—a tube placed in a large vein in the arm, neck, or groin that's used to give fluids. They can use thrombolytics to dissolve a blood clot. They can administer nitroglycerin through an IV.

But now, we were putting a stopwatch on our efforts.

"So now it's twenty minutes?" one of the EMTs asked.

"Correct," I said. We were at roll call. "There are too many people out there who need our help," I went on. "If they're in asystole, twenty minutes is all we've got. When the clock runs out, you stop. One note— this applies to patients who are eighteen or older."

The EMT sighed. "What about the families?" she asked. "We're supposed to just turn around and tell them, *Sorry, time's up. Gotta go*?"

Like all the other EMTs and paramedics, every day she faced families who were desperate for her to do more, who insisted—like the Asian kid in Bay Ridge—that she take their loved one to the hospital.

Now, if a patient didn't come back after twenty minutes, the family would never know whether their loved one might have been saved.

"I can't keep track," the EMT said. She shook her head. "When will they stop changing the rules?"

When it came to PPE, the department kept lowering its standards. First, we were told to wear N95 masks to all calls. Then we were told to wear N95 masks only for patients suspected of having COVID. That was ridiculous. Every patient we treated was suspected of having COVID—we even had patients we'd picked up at car accidents who had signs of the disease.

The logical thing was to wear an N95 to every call and discard it. But we were responding to thousands of calls a day, which meant thousands of masks. We didn't have the supplies. So the FDNY had another bright idea: we should reuse masks.

It was like telling someone to reuse a condom. N95s are intended for single use. The New York State Health Department policy was to throw them away after each patient. But that's what I heard on a call in April with Chief Bonsignore; Dr. David Prezant, chief medical officer for the FDNY; John Sudnik, chief of department for the FDNY; and the leaders of Local 3261 and Local 2507. The Centers for Disease Control and Prevention said that you could reuse the N95, Dr. Prezant said.

Really? I thought. *The same CDC that said it was safe to breathe the air at Ground Zero?* I was not convinced. Sure, there are ways to decontaminate an N95 mask: You can dry it at 70 degrees or use vaporized hydrogen peroxide or ultraviolet light. But decontamination takes time and supplies. We had neither.

"Chief Bonsignore," I said. "You're the chief medical officer of EMS. You know that the department has always told us that the mask is single use only, right? But because the department wasn't prepared for the pandemic, you want me to go and tell my members, *No, it's okay. You can reuse the mask*? That will go over like a fart in church."

Silence.

"We won't do it," said Mike Greco, the vice president of Local 2507 and the guy who'd come to Elmhurst with me that day in March. "We are going to tell the members that if they don't have a clean mask, they are not going out."

. . .

A week after I heard the news of Greg's death, Mike Sullivan called. He'd seen an interview I did with Al Jazeera. After my interview on CNN, I got calls from a lot of media outlets. I'd done interviews with the BBC, Fox News, the *Daily News,* the *New York Post.*

"How you doing?" I asked. Mike and I had been checking in with each other every day by text, but we didn't always have time to speak. Between work, washing your uniform every day, trying to get food in the house, and sleeping for a few hours, there wasn't a lot of time for phone calls. "What did you think of the Al Jazeera piece?"

"It was great, Anthony. You've got the hang of this media stuff," Mike said.

Then he added, "But I think you should be careful, man. You don't want to be out there all the time."

"Why not?"

"I just worry. You're emotionally fragile. You're investing so much of your soul in this fight with the department. And the energy of the fight—it's overwhelming. And I think you should be careful about being the only one," he went on. "There's a threshold. When one person becomes the face of something, people begin to tune out."

"But Mike, there's only a few of us who can do it," I said. Vinny Variale, the president of my union, gave news interviews. We gave them in our capacity as union reps. But regular EMTs and paramedics didn't have that cover. "Other people don't want to stick their necks out. I get it."

I wasn't trying to hog the spotlight. I was just trying to get the word out. And it seemed to be working. We'd gotten more help—food, masks, mental-health support, donations to the EMS FDNY Help Fund. We received letters at the station thanking us for our work. That popular support didn't translate into better pay and benefits, but when the time came to negotiate with the city, it would make it harder for officials to say no. Or so I hoped.

"Do you want to do some media?" I asked. Mike was very articulate and telegenic. "You'd be great at this."

"I'm not gonna do it," Mike said. "You're driven by the fight. I appreciate that. But I don't have that fight in me anymore."

It was true. Mike and I were yin and yang. I was out there with my fists flying; Mike was doing his job—a very important job—and trying to stay out of the fray. Some ALS coordinators, like the one who'd made it to the apartment near Green-Wood Cemetery just after we pronounced the patient dead on April 5, had gone back to working on an ambulance. My friend Sara Lupin, the paramedic with the special rescue unit, was asking to be put on COVID calls. But Mike had opted to keep working at his desk. He had no desire to return to the trenches. Not because he was afraid of getting COVID. He assumed from the start that we'd all be infected eventually. He just didn't know how much of the city's suffering he could take.

"I don't feel that I need to be a hero on the street," he told me. "I don't want to carry the pain, the sadness, the loneliness, the fear and the anger that keeps getting on us."

Mike's voice was weary. "I've seen enough."

MAY 2020

He's around back."

The man led us along the side of the house. Thin man, thin mustache. Dark eyebrows. It was early May. The rush of hospitalizations and deaths was tailing off dramatically. The number of people being hospitalized each day was less than a fifth of what it had been a month earlier, and the number of people dying every day had dropped below three hundred. Only two months ago, these numbers would have made a person's hair stand on end, but after April they were cause for relief.

Still, we continued to pick up one COVID patient after the next. Now I was with a hospital paramedic crew in Bensonhurst, not far from Villabate Alba, the pastry shop where I'd bumped into Joe in September, which now seemed like a lifetime ago.

The man's home looked spacious—three floors. There was a yard at the front with a chain-link fence. It had flower beds, but nothing was growing. We walked down a concrete driveway to a garage with a roll-up door. Beige vinyl siding.

As we walked, the man said, "My father's not doing so well. He's having trouble breathing." When we reached the garage, the man gestured to a small door. "Go ahead," he said.

He stood aside to let us pass. The crew and I looked at one another. We were puzzled. Then we pushed open the door, and I followed the medics inside.

The garage was gloomy. A 40-watt bulb hung from a cable in the ceiling. There were windows down one side, but they were grubby and didn't let a lot of light in. There was a refrigerator in the far corner. It made a low hum.

To the right of the fridge was a foldout cot with springs and a metal frame, the kind they give you in a hotel when you ask for an extra bed. There was a table next to it. A man lay on his side on the cot, covered by a red blanket. He turned over as we came in.

I looked around the garage. Tools hung on one wall: shears, a vise, an orange hacksaw. There was a stack of white plastic garden chairs, a table piled with cardboard boxes, an old moped. Near the bed was an electric radiator. The walls were unfinished. The studs were exposed. There was no insulation.

I wondered whether the radiator could warm the whole room. The days were mild, but the temperature still dropped at night. "Jesus," I mumbled.

One of the medics settled next to the cot. She took out her blood pressure cuff and a stethoscope. The man said his name was George. He was seventy-four.

"Nice to meet you, George," she said. "How are you doing? Can you tell us what's going on with you?"

George was breathing with difficulty. He said he was getting crazy fevers. Sweating.

"Are you receiving treatment for any medical conditions?"

"I'm diabetic," George said. "I have high blood pressure."

The medic had George lie quietly while she checked his blood pressure. She put a pulse oximeter on his finger. She palpated his stomach, checked his conjunctiva. His oxygen saturation was in the eighties. By pandemic standards, that wasn't too low.

I stepped outside.

"How long has your father been out here?" I asked the son.

About a week, the son said.

"Why are you keeping him like this?" I said. This was outrageous. After this, we'd fill out an elder-abuse form and send it to adult protective services.

"He wasn't feeling good, so we took him to the clinic," the son said. As he spoke, he avoided my eyes. "He tested positive. We needed to keep him away from the family."

I glanced up at the house. *Such a big place,* I thought. *There's got to be a room up there your father could stay in.* And I didn't buy the bit about the son taking him to the clinic. A man who would store his sick father in the garage didn't strike me as the kind of guy who would take him to see a doctor first.

"Where does he go to the bathroom?" I asked. "How does he bathe?" The son didn't answer my questions.

"We check on him" was what he said. "We check on him all the time."

The medics inserted an IV. The guy was dehydrated, and if he started to crash, he might need medication. They put a nonrebreather mask on him to give him some extra oxygen. I'd seen sicker COVID patients, but I would have taken George to the hospital even if he'd had no symptoms. We couldn't leave him in the garage with the hacksaw and the fertilizer. I was livid.

We wheeled him out to the ambulance. Once we shut the back doors, I turned to the medic who was driving. "Were you ever here before for this guy?"

"No, Lou. Never seen him," he said.

"Can you fucking believe it?" I said. "Putting your dad in the garage?"

"It's crazy," the medic said. "Everything is nuts. Nobody knows what they're doing right now."

It wasn't the first time I'd seen something like this. The man in the garage reminded me of a call I'd gone on a few weeks earlier to an apartment building near Station 40. When the crew and I arrived, there was a bed in the hallway, outside the apartment. We almost tripped over it.

The patient was an elderly Latina. She didn't speak English. She was propped up on some pillows, coughing and feverish.

Her daughter stood by the door of the apartment.

"What's she doing out here?" I asked.

"She's sick," the woman said. The rest of the family was in the apartment, she said. The grandmother didn't have her own bedroom. They didn't know what to do with her. "We wanted to isolate her."

"But she's not isolated," I said. We were on the fourth floor of an apartment building in Sunset Park. There were four apartments on each floor. "She's in a hallway. This is a common area. All the families who live on this floor—your mother could make them sick."

The idea that each time this woman left her apartment, she saw her sick mother was screwed up. The idea that the old lady slept alone in the hallway at night was shocking.

"Do you understand how this virus works?" I asked. "You can't leave her out here."

As we loaded the sick woman into the ambulance, one of the EMTs told me that she'd thought at first that the family had wheeled the grandmother out into the hall to make our job easier. The EMT had made a very generous leap of logic. She had given the family too much credit.

Other than episodes like the grandmother in the hallway, the battle with the pandemic took place behind closed doors: inside hospital rooms, inside people's homes, inside a racing ambulance. A city that used to live on the streets had shut itself away. People worked on Zoom. They ordered takeout from Seamless. They watched Netflix. Families stood on sidewalks and held up messages for their relatives to see: WE LOVE YOU. WE MISS YOU.

For months, no one went into anyone else's home. No one but first responders.

We went from one apartment to the next, from nursing home to nursing home. We saw what pandemic life looked like in people's bedrooms and living rooms. We saw the kids crowded around the laptop. We saw families consumed by fear. We walked into households where everybody was sick, where it seemed like a dark angel had passed over them. We watched patients say goodbye to their families before we drove them to a hospital that they might never leave.

We saw how the deck was stacked against the poor. The poor were more likely to work in jobs where they had contact with the virus, more likely to have health complications that made the virus deadly, more likely to live in a situation where social distancing was impossible. It's one thing to isolate yourself when you have a spare bedroom and two bathrooms. It's a different thing when five people sleep in the bedroom and four more sleep in the living room. Or when people share a bed in shifts, one sleeping while the other works.

Everywhere we went, we saw the efforts that people were making to shield themselves from the virus. They turned closets into sleeping capsules. They slept in unfinished basements. They hung plastic-strip curtains, like the ones used in meat lockers, across the entrances to their bedrooms. They rolled up towels and put them along the cracks at the bottom of the doors as if the virus were a draft that they could keep out.

We strode like apparitions into these terrified families' homes. We were gowned and masked and wore goggles that made us look like laboratory techs. One of my most powerful tools as an emergency medical worker is the ability to connect with people. I can reassure them, offer comfort when they are scared or grieving, coax them into accepting care. But now, I didn't even look human. My eyes were covered. My mouth was covered. I was like Charon the ferryman in Greek mythology, waiting to take them across the river Styx and into the world of the dead.

When families couldn't isolate sick relatives, they all got infected. Again and again, we went to a house to deal with an elderly COVID patient and found that his or her spouse had died days earlier.

There was that woman in Sunset Park who'd lost both parents days apart. There was a bedridden man in Bensonhurst whose wife was sick with COVID; she'd gone into cardiac arrest and died. The family called a few days later, one of the medics told me, and an ambulance had gone to the house. Same bedroom—now the husband was dead.

There was the elderly woman in Bay Ridge who lay next to the body of her husband as dependent lividity spread across his back and the backs of his legs. Northmore had to explain to her that her husband was gone. The woman's blood pressure was low and she most likely had COVID too, Northmore thought. But she refused to go to the hospital. So Northmore made her some buttered toast, fetched her a glass of water, and waited with her for the cop who would take custody of her husband's body.

There were times when families' efforts to shield themselves were so desperate, it was heartbreaking to witness.

A week or so after I found the patient in the garage, I went to the house of a Middle Eastern family who had tried to turn their sick elderly mother's room into a makeshift ICU. A man in his forties—the patient's son—showed me upstairs and to the bedroom. The family members had gowns and gloves that they wore when they cared for her. They had hung plastic sheeting around the bed in the shape of an *L*. It looked like they had taken translucent shower curtains and joined them together.

Behind the curtain lay a woman in her seventies. She was sucking air, using accessory muscles to breathe—intercostal muscles, the trapezius muscles in the upper back and shoulders. The hollow in her throat deepened every time she took a breath. That's called tracheal tugging, and it happens when your diaphragm is working extremely hard to help you breathe.

Two medics were with her getting a three-lead EKG. She had a pulse oximeter on her finger. The patient was obtunded, meaning she was conscious but she wasn't responding to anything the medics said; she moved only when the medics tapped her shoulder sharply.

"What's up, guys?" I said. They looked at me. One of them gave a slight shake of the head that meant that we were going to have to intubate the patient. Her oxygen saturation level was around 60 percent. Her blood pressure was extremely low. I set up the supplies we needed while the medics sedated the patient. Then one of them tried to insert the breathing tube. Once. Twice. He was having trouble.

I asked if I could take a look. That's a delicate thing—as a lieutenant, I try to avoid interfering with medics' patient care.

"Go for it," he said.

I looked down the patient's throat. Her spine was extremely hunched, a condition called kyphosis that's common in the elderly. As a result, her anatomy was squished to one side. I couldn't see directly down her throat.

"Can you pass me a six-millimeter?" I asked. We had been using a 7.5 millimeter endotracheal tube.

Bingo. We got it in.

As we carried the woman to the ambulance, the son followed us out. "Can I please come with my mother?" he asked.

"I'm sorry," I said. "We're not transporting family members. The hospital won't let you in." Her oxygen level had gone up slightly. She was now at 68 percent. But it still didn't look good. "Your mother is very, very sick," I told him. "I promise we're going to do everything we can. The hospital will do everything they can too."

"I can't let her go," the son said. "Please. Can't I just come? I know I could catch COVID. But I can't let her go like this."

He was on the edge of tears.

"Look, the only thing you can do is follow the ambulance to the hospital," I said. "It's not far. But you won't be allowed in. I'm sorry. I know this is very hard."

The man stood at the end of the stretcher. His mother was unconscious. Intubated. We didn't know this yet, but she wouldn't even make it to the hospital alive.

"Mom, we'll see you soon," the man said quietly. "These people are going to take care of you. I love you," he added. He held her feet as he spoke. He lingered for a moment. Then we gently rolled his mother into the ambulance.

At the end of the first week of May, I had an unexpected chance to talk about what it was like to walk into the homes of people suffering from the virus. And about the way that the pandemic had affected first responders.

I was invited to participate in a panel discussion of *Oedipus the King* by Sophocles. The event was part of a project called Theater of War run by a guy named Bryan Doerries. Bryan is an incredibly thoughtful man and a great listener. He translates Greek tragedies, and he puts on performances for military families and others who are suffering trauma.

On this occasion, a group of actors would read sections of *Oedipus,* then the panel—an emergency medicine doctor, the leader of an Asian-American advocacy group, a grassroots organizer, and I—would talk about how the play related to their experiences. And the audience would join the discussion.

The actor Jeffrey Wright had put my name forward for the panel. We met during the pandemic. Wright had set up a GoFundMe called Brooklyn for Life! to buy meals for health workers, and he started donating food to the staff at the Brooklyn Hospital Center in Fort Greene. Then he added other medical facilities and EMS stations. His organization dished out thousands of meals every day, and I was his point of contact when he set up the food deliveries for EMS. Jeffrey was reading the part of Tiresias, a blind prophet. When Bryan was looking for a health-care worker for his panel, Jeffrey suggested me.

The performance took place on Zoom. No props. The actors were in their living rooms. Frances McDormand played Jocasta, the mom (and wife) of Oedipus. She looked very pale and ghostly.

I was amazed by how much a play that's twenty-five hundred years old could resonate in our time. There were so many parallels. For one, we had our own mad king in Donald Trump. And the wails and groans of the city of Thebes that Oedipus describes—New York had those too: the cries of the sick and the endless ambulance sirens. Plus, the characters in the play see only what they want to see; they ignore what they don't like.

Tiresias, the blind guy played by Wright, tells Oedipus that he's the one who's truly blind. "You cannot see the evil that surrounds you, the iniquity in your home," he says.

Tiresias could have been talking to us New Yorkers. We pretend that we're so progressive, that we're living in a society built on equality and opportunity, but it's a myth. The pandemic revealed that.

Oedipus and his uncle bicker while the city is being devastated by a terrible pestilence. Like Trump and Cuomo. Like Cuomo and de Blasio—they couldn't even agree about the death toll in the city.

Jocasta loses it with them. "There are people suffering out there," she says. "Dying of the hateful plague. And this is what you choose to do with your time?"

Our politicians were sniping at one another, and the virus was still darkening the city, but some of our coworkers had recovered. Kenny was back. Jimmy was back. Juan Rios was out of the hospital and convalescing at home. We were still shorthanded, but it wasn't as bad as it had been a couple of weeks earlier.

Then Joe Marino got sick. He couldn't believe it. Joe was in his twenties. He worked out. He took pride in the fact he'd avoided the virus. But Joe had been doing double duty during the pandemic. In addition to being an EMT, he was a mortician. It was his family's business. So Joe had been treating patients on an ambulance and then preparing the dead for burial. First responder, last responder, as Arnold Chen put it. How Joe kept his shit together is a mystery.

He hadn't gotten COVID, though. Until now. So while we were happy to be reunited with our recovered colleagues, his case was a reminder: we were not out of the woods.

As our own EMS workers returned to the front lines, some of the out-of-town crews went home. Their help had been crucial to us. They'd taken a load off our shoulders when it mattered most, and we were willing to do the same for them if and when the time came.

They'd also been a breath of fresh air at a time when life was distinctly claustrophobic.

One afternoon, not long after the FEMA reinforcements had arrived, a pair of burly white men had knocked on the door of the station. I was sitting the desk or maybe picking up supplies; I don't recall. Outside, they had parked a blue and white ambulance. Not a New York City ambulance.

"Come in," I said. The guys were huge and pale. They looked more like farmers than EMTs. "Don't sit out there in your ambulance," I said. "Make yourselves at home here. We have coffee. We have food."

Thanks to people like Jose Rosario, we had plenty to eat. Charitable organizations as well as residents in the neighborhood kept dropping off food. We had a constant supply of doughnuts, pizza, muffins, jerk chicken, croissants, sandwiches, Thai curries. Many of us were starting to pack on what health-care workers called the COVID pounds.

"Where you guys from?" I asked.

"Minot," one of them said. "North Dakota."

I imagine they expected me to say, *Where?* Or just look at them with a blank expression. Minot is a small town in the middle of a huge prairie.

"I've been to Minot!" I said.

"For real?"

For real. I'd spent a night in a hotel in Minot years ago when I was driving to New York from Bozeman, Montana. The winters there are terrible, and it was freezing. I went to a bar next door to the hotel. It was a strip club, full of biker types and girls in cages. I stood out like a sore thumb. I got to talking to a girl, and her boyfriend became jealous and started getting in my face. There was some pushing and shoving. I realized I was outnumbered and I ran. Out of the bar and down the street, with five big guys chasing after me.

"Well, that sounds like Minot," one of the EMTs said.

I thanked them for coming so far to help us. We talked about the pandemic, how crazy it had been. "First time in New York?" I asked.

"Sure is. We drove to Times Square," one of the EMTs said. "Didn't see a soul."

"It's like that Will Smith movie," said his partner. "The one where the virus wipes everybody out. And he's walking around New York with his dog," he went on. "And there's nobody."

In addition to the guys from Minot, we had an overnight crew from Los Angeles who came and hung out at the station, a man and a woman in their twenties, both Latino. They walked around wide-eyed. They took the subway during the day and rode all over the city. They couldn't believe how dense it was compared to the sprawl of LA, how you could go ten blocks and be in a different country.

I was impressed by the pair of them. Sure, when I was twenty-three, I was off having adventures in Montana. But I wasn't driving around an unfamiliar city and walking into strangers' homes in the middle of a pandemic. That took guts.

At the same time, those two kids made me think about the problems that exist in EMS at a national level. We were in a city where a thousand people were dying every day. You'd think they'd send the EMS equivalent of Navy SEALs, people with chiseled features who could hold their breath underwater for an hour. But instead, they sent a couple of kids.

As work slowed down and colleagues returned to the station, I felt it was time to let loose a little. My birthday is May 12. For me, there's a melancholy to this time of year because Richie died soon after my birthday, my dad's birthday was two days before mine, and my nephew Eddie died in May. But I always celebrate—take a short trip, go to a concert. There'd be no travel or concerts this year, but we could get the Group Home together, at least.

Angie planned a party for me. She and Mike organized it at the house of our friend Raj, who lives in Queens. They hung green and white streamers in the living room and put up photos of me and the Group Home friends on our travels: My head poking out of the lavender in New Zealand. Me standing next to a lake in Acadia National Park in Maine.

There were more than a dozen of us. It was the first time we'd gotten together as a group since the virus hit. We'd hung out in twos or threes from time to time, but we'd been working too hard to socialize much.

Most New Yorkers with any brains were still keeping their distance from one another at that point. They weren't going to parties or visiting friends in their homes. But for us, the horse was out of the barn. Some of us knew we had had COVID, and the rest of us figured there was a decent chance we'd had it but had been asymptomatic. And we spent our days in close quarters with one another and with patients in ambulances and inside people's homes. It just didn't make sense for us to social distance.

At the party, everyone was a bit high—not on alcohol or drugs but on being together celebrating something. We needed to let off steam. I drank a couple of gin and tonics too quickly. I'm not a big drinker, so I felt tipsy. Angie was also on the G and Ts. She was a lot more tipsy than me. She danced with Andres, the pretty boy of the group who we always tease. He tied his T-shirt in a knot to expose his six-pack, and he and Angie strutted around the living room like models on the runway.

It felt good, like we were exploding out of a cocoon. We took a group photo, all of us wearing little green crowns that Angie had bought for us. In the picture, I'm in the middle. I have a big goofy grin on my face.

At the end of the night, we sat on the back porch and smoked cigars. It felt like a normal evening. Almost.

There were other moments that felt a bit like old times. There was an afternoon in late May when I responded to a call from an elderly lady in Sunset Park. I think her name was Maria. She had a Puerto Rican flag hung above the mantel, so I assume that's where she was from. The mantel was covered with tchotchkes. Little penguins, a coqui (the tiny brown frog that's native to the island and that I saw in droves when I visited).

An EMT crew had checked Maria's vitals and wanted to transport her, but Maria had refused to go. So I'd come to back up the EMT crew.

Maria was seventy-eight years old. She'd had a steady fever. She appeared to have pneumonia. It can be hard to distinguish pneumonia from COVID, but the woman's fever wasn't spiking up high, and her lungs sounded a little wet, which is typical of pneumonia.

"Maria, we need to take you to the hospital," I said. "We need to do some tests to see what's going on with your lungs."

But Maria was afraid that she would catch COVID in the hospital. She hadn't left the apartment in weeks, she said. She didn't allow visitors.

"I'm fine right here," Maria insisted.

"You need antibiotics," I said. "I'm afraid that we can't leave you at home."

As I spoke, I glanced at the coqui. The frog can survive off the island, but only in places with a similar habitat. *This elderly woman doesn't want to leave her habitat,* I thought. I'd seen that many times. Old people want to hold on to their independence. They're afraid to go to the hospital because they think they will die there.

"How do you know I won't get the virus?" Maria asked.

"The crew will protect you," I said. "The hospitals aren't like they were earlier in the spring."

There was a pause. Then Maria said, "I'll go if you'll help me with something. Can you put on my wig?"

"Sure," I said, smiling. "I don't think I've ever put a wig on someone, but I'm happy to try."

Maria had a scarf tied around her head. She took it off. She was bald. She pointed to a wig that was sitting on a bust on the dresser in her room. It was salt-and-pepper and wavy.

"Take that tape," she said. I picked up a roll of skin-colored tape that was beside the wig. "You need to make a cross on my head with the tape."

I stuck the tape to her crown, then placed the wig on it. "There," I said.

Maria reached for a hand mirror. "It's on backward," she said.

"Sorry, Maria," I said. "It's not like I do this every day."

"Hold the mirror," said Maria.

I took the mirror, and Maria removed the wig, turned it around, and put it back on. She looked at herself. She turned her head to one side, then the other.

"That's good," she said. "I'm ready to go."

As I walked with Maria to the door of her apartment, I felt a little wave of comfort. These brief exchanges with patients—the moments of connection—were what I'd always enjoyed. And I'd missed them these past two months.

Helping Maria with her wig also drew my mind back to something I had done years earlier for my father.

In 2012, two days before Dad died, I flew down to Florida to see him in hospice. He'd had liver failure and gotten a liver transplant, but now his transplanted liver was failing too. He was very weak and lethargic because his liver wasn't getting rid of certain toxins, like ammonia, and they were building up in his bloodstream. He looked like a mess.

Dad had been living in Florida for several years with a woman. She'd seemed nice enough at first but turned out to be an unhappy drunk.

Still, Dad and I had grown less distant. I'd pulled away from him after Richie died. I was pissed off at him for abandoning us and for letting Richie fail. And I'd wanted nothing to do with his junkie girlfriend. *You didn't have time for your son when he was on drugs,* I thought, *but you have time for her?*

As the years passed, though, we became closer. When Mom moved in with Dad in Philly, I started to see him more often. Our feelings were less raw. We'd gotten to a stage where we were comfortably numb.

When he moved to Florida, I visited him from time to time. He lived in a fifty-five-and-older community. Pool, palm trees. Part of me was glad he'd found a place to be peaceful and part of me resented it.

Now Dad was approaching the end. After sizing up his condition, I asked the nurses to give him an extra dose of lactulose, which decreases ammonia levels in the blood. Then I went out and bought some rum raisin ice cream, Dad's favorite flavor. I had to drive twenty miles each way to fetch it. I also bought a razor and some pomade.

When I returned to the hospital, I sat Dad up in bed and shaved him. I smoothed his hair. I fetched his teeth from the bathroom, and he put them in.

"How do I look?" he said.

I told him, "Dad, you're good to go."

I brought him a mirror. He held it up.

"That's nice, Anthony," he said. "Thank you."

By the end of May, the EMTs and paramedics at my station were starting to get used to the smoother pace. They were catching up on sleep, getting a day off here and there. Daily deaths from COVID-19 were in the double digits for the first time since the third week of March and only a few people were being hospitalized each day. We'd climbed the mountain and now we were coming down the other side—or so we hoped.

The surgery on my arm was put off yet again. Now I had no idea when it would happen. But I was resigned. So many people had had to postpone more urgent surgeries than mine. I'd gone this long; I could get by for a few more months.

EMS unions had convinced the department to shift to a twelve-hour rotation. That meant two tours—or shifts—per day instead of three. The logic of this was that you could split the station in two, and half the station would rarely see the other half, which cut the risk of infection. It also made for a better schedule; we were guaranteed every other weekend off, and we could no longer be asked to work sixteen-hour days. You can't work a double when each tour is twelve hours long. Things were beginning to feel a little more manageable.

And then everything went crazy. Again.

On May 25 in Minneapolis, a white police officer named Derek Chauvin killed an unarmed Black man named George Floyd by kneeling on his neck for more than nine minutes. Protests broke out in Minneapolis, then spread to other cities. In New York, they started out peacefully but turned violent at night. Police beat protesters with batons. They sprayed them with pepper spray. Protesters torched police vehicles and threw bottles and bricks—or airmail, as we call it in the emergency services.

Only a few weeks had passed since the mayhem of April. EMTs and paramedics needed time to regroup, but a stupid cop in Minnesota had killed a man in the most violent and cold-blooded way imaginable, so here we were. In addition to the mask, the gloves, and the goggles, we each had to wear a bulletproof vest and an orange helmet.

EMS wasn't a target, but protests tend to be chaotic. In their blue uniforms and bulletproof vests, EMTs and paramedics could be mistaken for cops. And when people are riled up, they don't always differentiate. Any uniformed officer becomes game. An FDNY paramedic in the Bronx watched protesters take baseball bats to her ambulance. They threw bricks at ambulances in Manhattan. It was jarring. As an EMT or a medic in these protests, you had to worry about getting hit by airmail or tear-gassed or having a protester attack you or your vehicle. And at the same time—if you were me, anyway—you shared some of the protesters' anger and sense of injustice.

Emotions about Black Lives Matter ran pretty high in EMS. FDNY EMS is two-thirds nonwhite and almost half female. For a lot of members, especially Black members, the protests and the movement were very personal. They identified with Breonna Taylor, a woman in Louisville, Kentucky, who had been shot dead in March 2020 when police officers barged into her house in the middle of the night. Breonna was Black. She was an emergency department technician. She was twenty-six. There are plenty of people in FDNY EMS who could imagine themselves in her shoes.

As a lieutenant, I had to remind the crews to put politics aside.

"Listen up. There are going to be more marches today." It was roll call, late May. Now protests were top of the agenda. "Around Grand Army Plaza. If you need to respond in this area, go carefully. If you get drawn into a protest, try to respond with a PD unit." In other words, make sure that there's a cop nearby, just in case.

Just a month earlier, lieutenants had been keeping members up to speed on which hospitals were on diversion and going through the latest protocols for cardiac arrest. Now we were telling the crews to check their bulletproof vests and explaining what to do if they found themselves on a dead-end street. (Turn around and get out; you never want to be on a street without egress.) Everyone had questions: *Do I wear the N95 and the helmet? What if these people have COVID? Isn't this going to be a massive super-spreader event? How will they know that we're not cops? Will they read what it says on the vest?*

"This is fucked up, man," one EMT said. "I need a break."

"I know. It's a lot," I said.

"Fucking protesters," another EMT said. "They'll need a cop someday. Then we'll see."

Like I said, EMS was diverse, which meant we had people who wanted to abolish the police and people whose parents were cops and firefighters. We had people who voted for Bernie Sanders and people who voted for Trump.

"Look, I know you all have opinions, and you have a right to express them," I said. "But respectfully. And if you get called to a protest, I don't ever want to hear that you didn't treat a cop or a protester because you didn't agree with them. You don't refuse to treat a human being because you don't like their politics. If you do that," I said, "you're on your own."

On Saturday, May 30, Kelly Quirke and her partner got caught up in the protests. They were parked in their ambulance on a side street in East Flatbush. They were surrounded by police and protesters. The protesters had set fire to a police van and then climbed on the roof of a Speedway gas station and started throwing bottles and bricks.

"What do I do, Lou?" Kelly sounded nervous but not panicked. She was less than two years out of the academy, in her early twenties. She'd just been through the busiest period in EMS history. She'd seen dozens of deaths. And now she was navigating a riot.

"Stay behind the police line," I said. "Move when they move. Keep your head on swivel and don't get out of the ambulance unless absolutely necessary. And do not hit the gas if you are surrounded!"

I wasn't thrilled about having two relatively green EMTs staffing an ambulance in the middle of a violent protest. Riyad, Kelly's partner, had been working on the ambulance for only a month before coronavirus hit. Between the two of them, they had roughly two years' experience.

In my fantasy EMS service, a newly qualified EMT would ride on the ambulance as a third crew member for six months with an EMT like Bones. At the end of that time, new EMTs would ride with me for a few days so they could get down with other crews. Buff some jobs. They wouldn't be allowed to ride with a partner until they could demonstrate that they had all the patient skills necessary. But in reality, we're always short-staffed, so we rush new recruits through their internships and let them fill out their own patient-skills tracking sheets. We don't have time to do it properly; we need to put them on ambulances.

I knew that Kelly and Riyad were cool customers. They'd done a remarkable job during the pandemic. But it wasn't fair to expect an EMT with eighteen months' experience to navigate a complicated situation like a protest. What if things turned really bad? Would they know what to do? Would they see trouble coming?

Kelly and Riyad had just dropped a patient at Kings County that afternoon when they were dispatched to a ten-thirteen—an officer in need—on Flatbush Avenue. A police officer had been injured by fireworks at a protest, they were told.

"Four-One Boy for the ten-thirteen on Flatbush Avenue and Tilden Avenue."

"Four-One Boy, ten-four. Sixty-three."

The call turned out to be a false alarm. But once the EMS chief coordinating response at the protest saw Kelly and Riyad, he wanted them to stay until things blew over, to stage the ambulance behind the police line.

Kelly and Riyad ended up working at the protest past midnight. Injured police. Injured protesters. More police than protesters, on account of their being behind the police line. One officer was hit in the head with a metal barricade, another by a flying brick.

At one point, Kelly and Riyad had four police officers in the back of the ambulance, all of them covered in pepper spray. Kelly walked from one to the next, pouring water over their faces. The police caught the water dripping from their chins in plastic garbage bags so that it wouldn't soak their uniforms.

As the protest advanced, the police line retreated. Kelly had to turn the ambulance around on a narrow street, back up, or find some other way out of there. But reversing for a block or doing a U-turn in an ambulance is no cakewalk even if you've been driving one for seventeen years like I had.

"Just find a safe spot," I told her. "Get a block or two away from the protest. Update Dispatch every time you're relocated. Call for help if you need to."

Around one a.m., another four police officers ended up in the back of Four-One Boy. Some had head injuries. There were too many to treat. Kelly went over the radio to get permission from the chief who was staged nearby.

"We can't hold any more patients," she said. Protocol stipulated no more than four patients in the back of an ambulance. "We're gonna take them over to Kings County."

The chief told her to go ahead and after that to go home. She and Riyad were supposed to clock out at ten p.m. If it hadn't been for all those cops who needed to be taken to the hospital, they might have been stuck there all night. After the spring from hell, it was turning into that kind of summer.

JUNE 2020

A few days after Kelly and Riyad were caught up in the protests in Flatbush, I was called to the Metropolitan Detention Center. A big beige and orange building, it's next to the old docks in Sunset Park where my father once worked, about ten blocks north of the park with the geese.

MDC is a notoriously troubled jail. In the winter of 2019, inmates froze for a week because of an electrical failure. They had no light and no heat. Some protested. They refused to eat. Reportedly, they were punished. The jail has suffered multiple scandals: sexual assault and rape by guards, corruption.

A paramedic crew from a South Brooklyn hospital arrived at MDC before I did. They started working on the patient, Jamel Floyd, who lay on the floor of a big common area in the center of the building. There was a TV, tables where inmates could play cards.

Floyd was in cardiac arrest. But it didn't sound as if that had anything to do with COVID. He'd had a seizure, the corrections officers said. They'd brought him from his cell into the common area.

Floyd was drenched.

"Why's he so wet?" I asked.

"He did that to himself."

"He did?" That sounded highly unlikely. Why would a man who didn't feel well pour water on himself? And if he was having a seizure, how would he even do that? Maybe they'd thrown water on him to bring him around? Something didn't add up. But I wasn't going to get into a debate with the corrections officers. It would only hold things up and it wouldn't do any good.

One of the medics started an IV. Gave Floyd a dose of epinephrine and sodium bicarbonate. They inserted a breathing tube.

"Let's dry him off," I said. We couldn't defibrillate a patient who was soaking wet. We grabbed some paper towels and dried off his chest.

"We're gonna transport him," I told the medics.

The two corrections officers glanced at each other. I got the feeling they'd assumed we would pronounce the guy right here. Perhaps they thought that would make things less complicated for them. But Floyd was thirty-five years old, and we didn't know what had caused the cardiac arrest. We could transport him even without a pulse. We were going to give it our best shot.

We had a stretcher with us. Getting in and out of the jail is no easy feat, so we'd made sure to bring everything we might need from the ambulance. We rushed Floyd to the loading dock at the back. A door opened; we stepped through. It closed behind us. The next door opened. A gate rose. It fell behind us. Another gate rose.

"Doesn't this all seem a little fugazi?" I asked the medics as we loaded the patient into the ambulance.

"Yep," one said. "Pretty shady."

"I mean, how does someone who is having a seizure get water all over himself? Where would he get that much water from? It had to be the officers."

Fugazi indeed.

We later learned that Jamel Floyd had been pepper-sprayed so extensively that he'd had a heart attack. The pepper spray in his cell was so thick that one of the corrections officers involved had thrown up.

The Floyd family sued the Federal Bureau of Prisons. It seems that Floyd was having a psychiatric episode and broke the window in his cell. Dozens of officers responded. They pepper-sprayed him in the cell. They placed him in a restraint chair. I don't know if he was still in the chair when the paramedic unit arrived. All I know is that he was soaked, and my guess is that they wanted to get rid of the traces of pepper spray. I figure they knew that they'd used unnecessary force and they wanted to cover their tracks.

No wonder the city was marching.

Those marches, though, were complex for EMS to navigate. We were neutral in our work. But as I said, we weren't neutral in our feelings. And sometimes those feeling burst out.

The day after Jamel Floyd was killed, an EMT named Taylor Varela jumped on the megaphone of the private medical transport vehicle she worked on and shouted her support for Black Lives Matter.

Varela was twenty-four. She and her partner were driving near the Barclays Center in Brooklyn. The Barclays Center was ground zero for the Brooklyn protests.

"Get home safe," she said. "Do not let up. Black Lives Matter. We fucking matter."

People put videos of Varela on Twitter. Of course they did. She was suspended. But that led to such an outcry that her employer re-instated her.

I get it—they didn't want her using her service vehicle to express her politics. But when you see so much social and racial injustice, it's hard to keep a poker face and get on with the job. I'm not a Fuck Tha Police person. I'm not a defunder. I work with cops all the time. Most of the cops I have encountered are decent people trying to do a difficult job.

But shooting an unarmed woman in her bed because of a no-knock warrant? Kneeling on a man's neck? Keeping a man in a choke hold till he dies? Drowning an incarcerated man in pepper spray? There's no question that the police need reforming, and I like to think that any good cop would agree.

Left to my own devices, I might not have joined the protests. I supported Black Lives Matter, but I was too worn out to get involved.

My good friend Mike Sullivan, however, was fired up and ready to protest. He was very committed to the movement. As a gay man who knew a lot of gay Black men—marginalized men in an already marginalized community—he identified strongly with the cause. I agreed to march with him.

We met on a Sunday in June on Fourteenth Street in Manhattan, ate some sandwiches, then joined the marchers heading south. It was hot, in the mid-eighties, and it felt even hotter in the throng. A New Orleans band played. People held signs.

BREONNA SHOULD BE HERE!
DEAR WHITE PEOPLE, WE SCREWED UP!

As we reached Washington Square Park, a cry rose above the crowd: "We need a medic!"

Mike looked at me. We weren't here as medics. We were here as protesters. I was wearing a T-shirt and Ray-Bans. Mike had on a floppy fishing hat and Keen sandals and a surgical mask. No bulletproof vest. No helmet.

"Is there a medical person anywhere?"

"C'mon," I said to Mike. Ever the buff.

We pushed through the crowd. A woman lay on the ground, semiconscious. She was talking but she wasn't making sense. She was hot to the touch. It looked like heat exhaustion. She was sweating, which was a good sign. If you have heatstroke, you stop sweating. That's when the trouble starts. You can no longer cool yourself down.

"Okay, let's get some space around her," Mike said.

"Hey," I said. "We're paramedics. FDNY. What happened?"

"We were walking and she started to feel dizzy," a woman said. Her friend, I assumed. "Then she passed out."

We sat the woman up a little and tilted her head forward. We grabbed a shirt that her friend was holding, soaked it in water, and wrapped it around her neck. Eventually she came around; she sat up and drank. We moved into a shady spot under a tree. The Sam Cooke song "A Change Is Gonna Come" blared from a speaker. We hung around for maybe fifteen minutes. She seemed better. "You need to keep her out of the sun," I told her friend. "Get her somewhere she can cool off."

They thanked us. Mike and I rejoined the march.

The BLM marches were energizing and draining at once. And as the adrenaline of the spring and the protests gave way to exhaustion, I started to crash. I think many of my colleagues did.

I was strung out. I lay in bed at night looking at the streetlight across from my apartment. I yearned to have someone there with me. I missed my girlfriend. Ex-girlfriend—whatever. We had never officially broken up, but at this point our relationship consisted of friendly text messages and not much more. When I woke in the night, I would imagine her next to me. If I could just reach out and take her hand, I thought, I'd go right back to sleep.

During the day, I drank Red Bull to try and shake off the fatigue. I'm not a coffee drinker, so normally I drink one can of Red Bull as part of my daily routine. But now I was drinking four. I craved sweets. When old-school medics need a boost—dehydrated, hungover—they'll get coworkers to put an IV in and give them a liter of fluid and an amp of D50 (25 grams of glucose in a 50-milliliter syringe). Works like a charm, apparently. But I prefer to get my sugar by mouth. I munched jelly beans. I bought Snapples and Twinkies on the way home from work. I snacked on the free food at the station. My weight crept up to 270. Then 275.

I tried to meditate, but it was hard to empty my mind. I knelt in front of my altar. I breathed. I focused on maintaining my posture. But my mind would dart to the pain of isolation. Or to my family. I was still angry with them. I felt they'd never had my back. I'd been left to navigate life on my own. And now I was navigating the pandemic and I didn't have anyone to help me.

When I meditate and it goes well, I feel my blood pressure drop. I feel my breathing slow down. I feel like I'm in a kind of blankness. And when I stop, I have a sense of peace.

But in a moment when meditation should have helped me, I couldn't do it. If I'd had the Buddha sitting next to me saying, *Anthony, kneel down again. Breathe,* maybe I'd have been able to concentrate. But as it was, my mind would race. Eventually, I stopped trying.

I sat the desk as much as possible. There, I had the companionship of my colleagues. Working alone in the command car had its advantages: I was autonomous, and there was less departmental bullshit to deal with. But it was also isolating. I went from call to call, worked with one crew, worked with another crew. I didn't have a partner the way I used to when I worked on an ambulance. No soul mate, either at work or at home.

Plus, I needed a break. I was on the road almost nonstop in March and April. I had been less careful with my arm during those crazy weeks, and even the long hours driving had taken a toll.

I was also emotionally spent. I no longer felt an adrenaline rush when a cardiac arrest came over the radio. Instead, I felt the energy drain from my body. The idea of pronouncing a person dead or dealing with another family hit by COVID made me go weak.

This was what Mike had warned me about. It was the reason he had spent the spring behind the desk. Mike's job was vital. But he had kept a bit of distance.

"I feel kind of bad about it," Mike had said. "But I don't want to carry the karmic dust that lands on you in EMS anymore. It doesn't come off very easily."

He was right. I had a good coating of karmic dust on me. And it was hard to brush it away.

I asked the other lieutenant on my tour, Alex Loutsky, if I could work the desk instead of being on the road. I was burned out, I told him. Alex—the medic who'd jumped on the radio when the first plane hit the World Trade Center—was good with it. He liked to be on the road.

I used to like it too, of course, but now, all the Red Bull in the world couldn't restore my spark.

I wasn't the only one struggling. As a union representative, I field concerns from lieutenants and captains at stations all over the city. During May and June, I woke each day to a stream of texts.

I'm sick. I'm running out of sick time. They denied my LODI claim.

Back then, if an EMS member caught COVID, it wasn't considered a line-of-duty injury, which allowed up to eighteen months of paid leave. That's since been rectified.

Hey, Anthony. My mom passed. She had COVID. We need $$ for the burial. Can u help?

Anthony, the chiefs are bugging out. They're trying to get blood from a stone.

Ant, the members are checked out. I can feel it. I don't know how to reach them.

EMTs and paramedics were getting upset and losing their temper for no reason. They were shouting at their kids. Snapping at their spouses. Drinking. Dave, a dispatcher, looked at a photo of his daughters on his phone at a stoplight one day and burst into tears.

Colleagues told me that they tossed and turned at night like I did. They talked in their sleep. They had nightmares and flashbacks. One of the EMTs said that her partner sometimes dozed off in the ambulance during their tour and yelled in her sleep. Northmore dreamed that he walked into the station, and the apparatus floor was lined with shelves constructed from two-by-fours and plywood. That's how the shelves in the refrigerated morgue trucks are built. In the dream, the shelves rose all the way up the walls, maybe twenty feet. They were stacked with bodies. Northmore started taking melatonin to help him regulate his sleep.

Not everyone talked about what was going on in their heads. EMS workers don't find it easy to show that they are vulnerable. We're supposed to be the rescuers. We're not supposed to need help. So we see terrible things and try to shrug them off. Domestic abuse, suicide—these are calls that we should process psychologically, that we should sit down and talk about with a counselor, especially given that EMS workers are statistically more likely to contemplate suicide or kill themselves than civilians. But instead, we get a sandwich and a Diet Coke and we're good to go.

After firefighters respond to a fire, they gather at the station to talk through the incident. It's called a hotwash. They go over their responses—what went well, what they could have done better. How they are all doing. Firefighters eat together and sleep at the station. They are a brotherhood. I think it's over the top—kind of incestuous—but it's good for morale.

In EMS, by contrast, we don't even return to the station between calls. We don't have as many opportunities to build camaraderie. I think it's one of the reasons that we are burned out. We treat a patient—or watch a patient die—and then park on a street corner and wait for the next one.

During the busiest days in March and April, EMS workers checked in with each other outside hospital emergency departments. I drove to the emergency bays and handed out water and told the crews to take five. That was our hotwash, and it wasn't enough.

FDNY EMS doesn't have a good system for helping members process difficult calls or stress. The FDNY has a peer counseling unit, but it's one person coordinating a rotating staff of EMS workers who get only sixteen hours of training. The people in the unit mean well, but they're not professionals. And they conduct the counseling sessions in uniform. What kind of confidentiality does that suggest? What happens if the member wants to talk about his or her drinking problem? And what if the counselor recommends a month of rehab? Firefighters have unlimited sick leave. They can go to rehab for as long as they need without using a single vacation day. EMS workers have only twelve precious days a year, so a few weeks in rehab would mean losing their entire vacation allowance.

EMS also has access to the FDNY Counseling Services Unit. Its staff can offer support and refer us to professionals. During the spring of 2020, many of us turned to them. Calls to the CSU hotline rose by more than a third between the middle of March and the end of June. A colleague at CSU told me that there was so much demand, they were just ignoring some calls.

We received a few awkward visits from the EMS chiefs. They popped into the station unannounced, stood six feet away from the members, and kept their masks on. It felt very stiff. We'd stopped wearing masks inside the station weeks before. We figured if we caught the virus, it would be from a patient or from the person we sat next to in an ambulance, not from walking past one another on the apparatus floor. Flawed logic, maybe, but it was how we saw things.

So when the chiefs visited in their masks, it underlined the gap in their experience of the pandemic. We were the battle-worn. They were the sheltered ones who were still uptight about catching the virus.

Besides, the chiefs brought camera people with them. It felt like a publicity stunt, a way to show they were rallying the troops. They told us how proud they were; they talked about planning. They didn't ask the members how they were doing. How their families were. How they were feeling. A medic from a different Brooklyn station texted me in the middle of a visit from Chief Bonsignore.

She's talking about fucking logistics, he wrote. We haven't heard from her in months. And this is the first thing she talks about?

For some, the pandemic was more than they could bear. On June 19, a Friday, I was smoking a cigar with Mike, Pete Borriello, and Terence Lau in Pete's backyard in Queens when my phone rang. It was Andres Segovia, the pretty boy who had danced with Angie at my birthday party.

Dre's voice was shaking. "Anthony, Matt Keene is dead," he said. "He killed himself."

Matthew Keene was a lieutenant paramedic at Station 17 in the Bronx. He was incredibly sweet-natured. Very popular with the crews. We all knew him. Mike and Angie knew him especially well. They'd worked in the Bronx for years.

Matt Keene wasn't the first. Two months before Matt killed himself, John Mondello, an EMT who worked for the FDNY in the Bronx, shot himself in the head on the banks of the East River. He was twenty-three. He had been out sick for a couple of days with what he believed was COVID.

I didn't know Mondello, but he had a reputation for being smart and cheerful. He had joined FDNY EMS two months before the pandemic hit. His friends told reporters that he found the chaos and the amount of death that they were witnessing very distressing, that the pandemic caused him a lot of anxiety. His mother told reporters that he felt he had been bullied at his station. I don't know if that was the case. What I do know is that no first responder, let alone a kid with two months on the job, should have to go through what we went through during the pandemic.

And now Matt was dead too.

During the spring of 2020, Matt had become isolated. He lived alone. His coworkers were his family, but he couldn't hang out with them like he had during non-pandemic times.

A couple of weeks earlier, Matt had called me about some trouble he was having at work. He was a union member. He had pushed back against a superior who was making life difficult for members of his station, and the superior had written him up for insubordination. All Matt wanted to do was protect his crews, and the department was giving him a hard time.

That Friday morning, Matt hadn't shown up for work, Dre said, so he'd gone to his apartment in Nyack. It's about twenty-five miles north of the city on the Hudson River. If a member doesn't show and doesn't call, our protocol is to check on them. Dre forced entry and found Matt in his bedroom with a gunshot wound in his head.

When I hung up the phone, Mike and Terence and Pete had fallen quiet. They were looking at me. I told them what had happened. Mike put his head back and gazed at the sky.

He muttered, "That poor soul."

I texted Angie to call me. Angie had been very close to Matt. She loved working with him. She'd been stationed in the Bronx until 2019 and she and Matthew had worked overtime together several days a week.

Angie knew that Matt suffered from depression. He was lonely and he wanted a girlfriend. He and I had connected on that level, at least.

After Angie moved to Brooklyn, she texted Matt constantly. If he wanted to get together, she always said yes, even if it meant using a sick day. She couldn't bear to let him down.

Angie called, and when I told her what had happened, she was silent. Then she said, "You're joking, right?"

"I'm not, Angie. I'm so sorry," I said.

I heard a choking sound. "I can't believe it," she cried. "I was just talking to him. Two days ago. I was just talking to him, Anthony."

Then she hung up.

Angie doesn't cry easily. She's not emotional like I am. But Matt's death crushed her. Matthew had always confided in her, she told me. Why hadn't he said anything?

A couple of days later, at work, Angie looked grim. "People keep asking me if I'm okay," she said. "It's such a stupid question."

"What do you tell them?" I asked.

"I tell them, *Well, I'm alive. I didn't kill myself.* Then they look at me like that's a fucked-up answer."

Angie kept a picture of Matt in her locker. She was angry. Not with Matt. But she was angry that what happened, happened.

I wanted to raise my colleagues' morale—and mine—so I started cooking for the station on Sundays. I hadn't cooked for months. We'd been too overworked to think about cooking in the spring, and nobody would have been comfortable sharing food.

But things were much slower in June, and cooking seemed like a good way to bring the crews together. Plus, I needed something positive to keep me occupied.

I started looking up recipes. If I included both the daytime tour and the crew that came in in the evening, I needed to feed at least twenty people. I spent ages thinking about what to make.

I texted Yvonne. Yvonne was a good cook and she wrote recipes down and held on to them. We'd been in contact every week since she'd reached out to me in March—texting, a phone call here and there. She checked in on me. She talked about her health. Yvonne worried about her health constantly. She was heavy and she had heart problems. We didn't get into anything deep or talk about what had kept us apart all this time. We didn't talk about Richie or my parents or even Eddie, who'd died at twenty-nine, the same age Richie was when he died. Still, it was good to be back in touch.

Can u send me the linguine salad recipe? I texted.

Sure. What's up?

I'm gonna cook for the station.

Cool.

Also the chicken Marsala?

I decided to start with Italian sandwiches with sausage and red peppers. I toasted the bread and let the mozzarella melt on top of it. I made a macaroni salad with onions and parsley and chopped egg. Even Joe Marino liked it, and Joe hated macaroni salad.

We sat in the yard at the back of the station. We had a table and chairs and a big red sunshade. Someone had a portable speaker. Joe had just responded to a call from Patricia, the hypochondriac in the big brick house. She had bought herself a pulse oximeter. Many people did during the pandemic because they'd learned that low blood oxygen was a key symptom of COVID. Now Patricia monitored her oxygen saturation constantly.

"She's like, 'My oxygen levels are going up and down,'" Joe said. "Then she walks up some steps and her oxygen goes from ninety-nine to ninety-eight. And then she says, 'See! My oxygen is falling.'"

"She's insane," said Kenny.

"Yep. But she didn't get COVID," I said.

"None of them did," said Kenny. "Somehow they all survived."

It was true; we were picking up the regulars again. They had disappeared during the pandemic. Some of them might have gone to the hotels where the city was housing the homeless, and some were probably passed to the FEMA crews since our ambulances were so busy. But now the regulars were back in our buses.

I'd picked up Maribel a week or so earlier. She'd complained to me that a john she'd slept with or done something sexual with had run off without paying.

"What are you doing getting so close to people, Maribel?" I said. "You need to be careful. You could catch the virus."

I was amazed that all the regulars appeared to have made it: Maribel. Classic Tile. The diabetic who was always drunk on the steps of Sunset Park.

Kenny had a theory. He figured that the frequent fliers had been exposed to so many germs, they had ironclad immune systems. "They're indestructible," he said.

If only we were too.

JULY 2020

Bones and I sat in the lounge at the station one afternoon in early July and watched reports on CNN about how COVID was ravaging America. Bones was eating a slice of pizza. He was on overtime.

The volume of calls to 911 was still low, so crews were spending more time at the station. They parked their ambulance outside, took a break to use the bathroom, grabbed a doughnut or a plate of chicken. Protocol demanded that crews return to their intersection—their eighty-nine—between calls, but the lieutenants were cutting them some slack. Nobody was about to get on anyone's case. We all needed company. And downtime.

New York was now in better shape than other parts of the United States in terms of COVID cases and deaths. During the first week of July, fewer than twenty people a day died of COVID-19 in New York City. The rate of infection statewide that week hovered around 1 percent. Testing was widespread because facilities—government-run and private—had popped up all over the state. The number of people taking PCR (polymerase chain reaction) tests each day in New York State was three times what it had been in April. In the spring, the lines to get tested were excruciatingly long, but the process had become straightforward. Which was lucky for EMS, since we still had to line up with everyone else.

The city had reopened little by little. Playgrounds were back in action. Restaurants were open for outdoor dining. Cuomo had permitted massage and tattoo parlors to open as long as they stuck to some social-distancing protocols.

Elsewhere, though, the picture was different. The virus had spread to almost every county of the United States and it was raging in other parts of the globe: Russia, India, Colombia, Indonesia, Nigeria, Peru. Brazil had recorded more than a million cases, and Brazilian president Jair Bolsonaro—a Trumpian idiot who was criminally dismissive of the virus—had tested positive.

Bones and I sat in the lounge together watching one COVID-related TV news report after the next. In the United States, the number of people who were hospitalized with COVID was as high as it had been in April, around sixty thousand. Americans were arguing about how much we should lock down and whether we should wear masks. Trump was still insisting that there was no need. He blamed the virus on the World Health Organization and pulled out of the group.

In Kentucky and North Carolina and Michigan and Texas and California, people protested stay-at-home orders. They worried about small businesses. They thought the lockdown violated their rights. *Their rights to do what?* I thought. *To get sick? To make other people sick?*

"This country is so off track," I said to Bones. I took a slice of pepperoni. "If you'd asked me a decade ago where the world would be in 2020, I'd have predicted that we'd have flying cars. Instead, we have a snake-oil salesman for a president and people who think it's an infringement on their rights if we ask them to wear a fucking mask."

"People are dumb, Anthony," Bones said. "Unfortunately, we can't treat them for that." Bones was reading something on his phone. "You see how much they're paying these tracers?" he said. "They're getting more than I am."

In New York City, the government was hiring hundreds of contact tracers. The tracers followed up with people who tested positive for

COVID-19 and tracked down people an infected person had been in touch with. They offered support to people who were infected. The job required "health-related professional experience" or public health training. The starting salary was $57,000, with benefits. More or less the same as a paramedic with several years of ambulance experience and a year of full-time school. The city was willing to pay something like a living wage to people who would collect data for them for a few months but not to the people who were tending the sick and getting sick themselves. Not that this was anything new. At the time, the New York City parks department paid its puppeteers better than the city paid many of its EMTs—a fact that was a running joke in EMS.

On TV, there was a news report about Texan hospitals running out of beds in the intensive care units. The state was reporting around eight thousand new cases a day. Hundreds of people had died. A record number had been hospitalized. They were heading into a tunnel very like the one we had gone through in March and April. But instead of tightening the lockdown, the Texas governor was allowing businesses to open. Texans could get their hair cut. They could go to water parks. They could go bowling and drink in bars.

Why are they keeping things open? I wondered. *Why didn't they listen to us?* New York got hammered by the virus. We had underestimated the disease. We had made mistakes. We should have shut down more quickly. But at least we had had an excuse. New York, Wuhan, Lombardy—these were the first places the virus caught fire. We didn't have all the information we needed; we didn't know how the virus spread, how it affected certain age groups. But Texas? California? Arizona? Florida? They'd seen everything that they needed to see. They'd watched New York and New Jersey burn. They'd heard the reports about nursing homes becoming death traps, about the graves on Hart Island in the Bronx, about the refrigerated trucks outside hospitals. What more did they need to know?

Bones looked at me. "I don't get it," he said. "Did they think that what we went through was a joke?"

"I don't know what to say, Al," I said. "I never thought that our country could end up in a mess like this."

The way people behaved—including some New Yorkers—was depressing. Most New Yorkers took the virus seriously. They wore masks to go jogging, to sit at an outdoor restaurant, to ride the subway. But even in EMS, there were people who doubted the danger of the virus.

People who hadn't caught the virus thought that they would never catch it. People who had caught the virus and recovered thought it was no big deal. There were first responders who still called it the "China virus," who said that Bill Gates was behind the pandemic and that he wanted to put microchips in us all. I didn't know what to say. These were health professionals. Where had they been working that spring? Had they been treating patients on another planet? Had they not seen what I'd seen, what Bones had seen?

What I saw at work each day didn't help my mood any. I was sitting the desk much of the time, but when I was on the road, I saw how the pandemic had wrecked people's lives. It left them scarred economically and psychologically. The impact of the virus was totally lopsided. It not only killed and sickened poor people and nonwhite people far more than it did other people, it also took their jobs.

We walked into homes where the refrigerator was empty except for some Ritz crackers and a half-full bottle of Pepsi. Homes where the table was piled with food from the food bank. We went on calls to apartments where nobody in the family seemed to be working. Everyone was home in the middle of the day. From what I could see, these weren't telecommuting, white-collar people. These were housekeepers and construction workers and office cleaners. Nearly one in five New Yorkers was without work in July 2020 and most of the jobs that had disappeared were in sectors where people didn't earn a lot to begin with—transportation, hotels, restaurants, movie theaters, stores. Those unemployed people were our patients.

And households had often lost more than one family member—two brothers; a mother and daughter. I am sure those families also had neighbors who'd died, friends who'd died. It was as if some zones of the city had been bombed while others hadn't been touched. The *New York Times* published a map showing that more than 40 percent of residents in Brooklyn's less expensive neighborhoods, like Borough Park, Brighton Beach, and Midwood—where I live—had antibodies to SARS-CoV-2, double the rate that was seen in wealthy sections of Brooklyn, like Park Slope.

Some people seemed to have lost so much—a parent, a job, the ability to pay rent—that they chose not to feel anymore. They shut down. This was as disturbing to me as the screaming and crying and bashing things that we saw when someone was overcome by loss. Outbursts like those are hard to witness, but they feel normal. That summer, though, I saw people who couldn't seem to muster any emotion. That was scary. Not least because I was starting to feel that way myself.

In July, I met a young woman in an apartment on Coney Island Avenue in South Brooklyn. Her mother had gone into cardiac arrest, and I was backing up a medic crew on the call.

It was a small apartment. The mother was on the floor of the living room. She was forty-six. There was a man in his thirties in the living room with the crew. He might have been a relative or a friend; I don't know. I remember him helping to move a table aside so that the crew could work on the woman.

The man said that the patient had been sick with a fever and a cough, typical COVID symptoms. He said another member of the family had died from the disease.

The young woman was in a small bedroom next to the living room. She sat in front of an old-fashioned wooden dressing table that had a circular mirror. She was applying eyeliner. She was very focused.

I stood in the doorway as the crew in the living room prepared to transport the patient. They hadn't gotten a pulse back, but they could continue CPR in the ambulance.

"You know, your mom is very sick," I said. "I'm afraid that she's not breathing. Her heart has stopped beating."

The young woman didn't stop what she was doing or turn and look at me.

"We're doing everything that we can," I said. "We're going to take her to the hospital."

The girl swiveled her chair around to face me. "Okay," she said. Then she turned back to the mirror, took out some lipstick, and started painting her mouth.

One morning not long after that encounter with the young woman, I got a flat tire on my way to work. It was around five thirty or maybe a little earlier. I'd barely slept, which seemed to be happening more often than not these days.

I had woken up at two in the morning. My mind bounced from one negative thought to the next. I'd stewed about the department and how it had let us down. About Greg Hodge and Matt Keene. I'd thought about my ex-girlfriend, about the time we'd spent all day in bed together. Recently, she'd told me that she was dating someone else. I was jealous. Resentful. It seemed that women wanted me when they had a crisis and dumped me the minute they were back on their feet. Now some other guy got to be with her, and I got *ungotzungool*—nothing.

I'd closed my eyes and tried to shut off my brain. I'd asked Siri to play soothing sounds—the sea or soft music. I started to drift off.

And then—*snap!*—I woke up again. I needed to pee. Once I was out of bed, I was wide awake. I scrolled through Twitter. I sent tweets to Nicole Malliotakis, a conservative nutjob who represented New York's Eleventh District in Congress. I read the latest on the Right Wing Watch website. Ever since my days listening to Rush Limbaugh in Montana, extreme right-wing politicians have provided me with fuel for my anger. Life was unfair. Women were unfair to me. My family was unfair to me. But it was easier to direct my ire at politicians.

At four, I got up and made myself some eggs. I had to be at work at six.

I had driven about twenty blocks when the tire-pressure warning light came on. I got out of the car and checked the wheels. The rear right tire looked a little low. *Shit,* I thought. I would be late. I hate to be late. I get everywhere on time.

Agitated, I called the station. Joe McWilliams picked up.

"I got a flat tire, Joe," I said. "I'm held up. I'm sorry, man."

"No worries, Ant," Joe said. "We'll see you when we see you."

I hung up. My pulse rate was high. *Stupid fucking tire,* I thought. I was going to be late for the first time in seventeen years.

I rolled into a self-service Mobil station on McDonald Avenue in Midwood, next to the big cemetery. Gas was just over two dollars a gallon—one of the few upsides of the pandemic. I filled the tire with air. I had a canister of sealant in the trunk. I squirted it into the tire.

I drove on. Pulled up outside the station. Already my phone was pinging. Messages from union members. Problems. Questions. I felt the pressure building in my chest. Why couldn't I get a break? Why was I here again, at six in the morning, busting a gut?

I turned off the engine and sat for a minute. Then I yelled at the top of my lungs. I pounded the steering wheel. I was a kid again, overwhelmed with frustration, shoving my hand through a glass door.

I don't know how long I yelled. Maybe it was a few seconds. Maybe it was a minute. My windows were rolled up. The air-conditioning was on. I hope nobody heard me.

I took some deep breaths, grabbed my keys and my phone, and headed into the station. It was a few minutes to six. I was still on time.

Being restricted to the city didn't help my gloomy mood. I hadn't left New York in six months, the longest uninterrupted time I'd spent in the city in seven years. Travel seemed risky, and many countries required visitors to quarantine upon arrival. New Yorkers were even required to quarantine if they visited Vermont!

I'm not one of those New Yorkers who have friends with houses upstate or on Long Island. And every house that an ordinary person could rent was booked. There just didn't seem to be anywhere to go.

I felt trapped. Travel is my oxygen. I travel the way that other people run obsessively or diet. It's fun, of course. But it's more than a pastime. It's part of a life that revolves around motion. I drive a fast vehicle when I'm working. I fly all over the world when I'm not. Hammerhead sharks have to keep swimming in order for oxygenated water to flow through their gills. They need movement to stay alive, and in a way, so do I.

One escape that I did have was my gig at Belmont Park on Long Island. In the summer, the races move from Aqueduct to Belmont. It's a gorgeous racetrack. Beautiful infield. Lots of trees. There's a grand old brick clubhouse covered in ivy. I worked there once a week. It wasn't stressful work, so it was like having a day in the country.

Belmont had opened in June but without the spectators, only jockeys and horses and the outriders who brought the horses to the starting gate. I was there for the jockeys and outriders.

One day in late July, I was at Belmont at dawn. The trainers take the horses out very early, and they have medics on hand just in case they fall. I was standing on the edge of the track when I saw a security guard I recognized from Aqueduct. He was the guy who called me when Sam, the old man, had been feeling sick in February. Sam, the World War II vet who had been going to Aqueduct for over seventy-five years. Who placed dime bets on the horses. Who lived alone. And who had worried about what he'd do if coronavirus closed down the track.

"Hey, bro! How you doing?" I asked the security guard. I didn't know his name, but whenever I saw someone from the days before the pandemic, I felt as if I were greeting an old friend.

"I'm good," the guy said.

We talked about the pandemic, how crazy it had been.

"Remember that old guy?" he said.

"The one who was watching the simulcast?" I said. "Sam? You seen him?"

"He got COVID," the guy said.

"You're kidding me."

Another of the security guards from Aqueduct had been in touch with Sam. Sam was such a regular at the track that the security guard had his phone number. In April, the guard called him and discovered that he was in the hospital with COVID. The guy checked on Sam by phone over the next couple of days. Then Sam stopped picking up. The guard called the hospital. Sam had died, the hospital said.

I thought of that old man alone in the hospital. I wondered if anyone other than the guard had checked on him. Whether anybody had claimed his body. There were hundreds of people being buried in the potter's field on Hart Island. Was Sam among them?

On July 30, I took part in another event put together by Bryan Doerries's theater organization. This time, instead of being on the panel, I had a small role in the play that was being discussed. I was the messenger in Sophocles's *Ajax*.

I was extremely excited. And extremely nervous. I would be reading alongside Amy Ryan and Chad Coleman. Finally! A decade after I let go of my Hollywood dreams, I would be onstage with two amazing actors. A Zoom stage, at least.

The week before the play, I printed out copies of the script. I got Angie and Jimmy to rehearse with me. We sat at the big table in the lounge at the station with our scripts in front of us, reading Sophocles aloud. It was surreal. Mike also helped out. We practiced over the phone, working on the tone, the inflections, and the rhythm of the lines. Mike was great; it was like being back in acting class.

Taking part in the performance was the highlight of the summer. It got me out of my world for a week, gave me something to think about that wasn't work and wasn't the pandemic.

But it's a dark play, and it resonated. Here's the plot: Ajax is angry because he has been denied the armor of Achilles. Ajax and Odysseus vied for it after Achilles was killed in battle, and Odysseus has been awarded the armor. Ajax feels like his sacrifice and bravery have not been acknowledged. He flies into a murderous rage.

Ajax's wife, Tecmessa, begs him not to do something drastic, not to abandon her and their child. Ajax pretends to take heed and says he's going to bury his sword.

Then the messenger arrives with instructions from a seer. Ajax must confine himself at home for the day in order to save himself from the wrath of Athena.

But the messenger is too late. Ajax has killed himself.

It's an ancient tale with goddesses who play tricks on mortals. But I related to it. To Ajax's frustration and sense of injustice, his temper, even his desire to end everything. Sometimes, during the months after the pandemic started, I felt the urge to tear things apart. I worried that the anger I felt at society, at the fire department, at the women who I believed had taken advantage of me, would come bursting out. I just didn't know how destructive I might be.

AUGUST 2020

A few days after I read in the Greek play, I was embroiled in a real-life crime drama.

I was in Canarsie, a middle-class Brooklyn suburb that's next to the water. A man in his twenties lay on a big brown sofa in the living room of a three-story story house. The house was very tidy, nicely kept. Turned out to belong to his mother.

The man was bleeding from a gunshot wound to his stomach. The bullet had entered his left flank and lodged itself in his abdomen. We couldn't find an exit wound, but he wasn't bleeding badly, and he wasn't vomiting—a good sign, since it meant that his stomach was probably intact.

Outside, half a dozen police cars were parked in the sun. Members of the Emergency Service Unit stood on the sidewalk. One of them talked into a radio handset. The ESU is a special operations unit. Its members wear black helmets, bulletproof vests. They must have been sweltering in those vests. A cop ran yellow incident tape around the edge of the front yard.

"They shot me!" the guy said from the sofa. He kept repeating this fact, as if anyone in the room were unaware of it. He spoke with a sing-song Caribbean accent. Trinidadian, I believe. "They shot me! Man, it hurts!" he cried.

It was early August. Elsewhere in the United States, the virus was still spreading. It was all over the South. It was in Texas. In California.

It was worsening in the Midwest. Between nine hundred and a thousand people were dying every day.

But in New York City and across the state, the virus had continued to recede. The daily death toll had fallen to single digits. The Black Lives Matter protests didn't seem to have increased infections. The number of new cases in the city was around three hundred a day—as low as it would be for many months.

People were still marching. I had been assigned to a few uneventful protests. A group of protesters camped outside City Hall and called on the mayor, Bill de Blasio, to reduce the budget for the police department and shift money from policing to youth services. He cut a billion dollars. On paper, anyway. He had a $9 billion deficit, so some of that money was bound to be taken from the NYPD.

And EMS was threatened too. De Blasio said he might have to cut four hundred jobs from the service. The city asked FDNY to supply the names of the four hundred newest EMS members. Firefighters, who outnumber members of the emergency medical services more than two to one, wouldn't be touched. Of course not. De Blasio was spineless; he bent himself double to please the fire department, did whatever it wanted. Which, of course, was to protect firefighters.

I was apoplectic. EMS went from being cheered at dusk to being threatened with pink slips in a matter of weeks. I got it; de Blasio was playing for federal funding or borrowing authority from Albany, the state capital. The city was in a huge financial hole. It had lost billions in sales tax and personal income and property taxes. New York City needed either a federal bailout or authority from the New York State legislature to issue long-term debt to cover its budget. But to use EMS members as pawns in a pissing match with the federal government or Albany was despicable.

If the city cut 10 percent of the EMS workforce, some people who needed an ambulance wouldn't get one. It was that simple. We were stretched to the breaking point already. And the people who wouldn't get an ambulance were the people in the city's poorest sectors—the same communities that had been hammered by the pandemic.

The day after we learned about the cuts, the *New York Post* published the salaries of the staff of Chirlane McCray, the mayor's wife. Her scheduler made more than a newly qualified paramedic. Her senior speechwriter made three times the starting salary of an EMT. This was the same First Lady who was in charge of the failing $850 million mental-health initiative called ThriveNYC. The program was supposed to target low-income patients who couldn't afford mental-health care and take on issues like drug abuse and suicide. If it worked, women like Maribel might get care and not have to ride in circles on the R train. But there was no accountability, and nobody seemed able to measure how effective the program was. The city was happy to waste taxpayer money on pet projects but didn't want to spend it on emergency health care.

The fact that the mayor dared to float job cuts in EMS told me a lot about our city. People put rainbows in windows to thank frontline workers, but they wouldn't stick up for us when it really counted. They turned on the solidarity when there was a crisis, then went back to living their lives.

And that's what they were doing now. The city, which only months earlier was in critical condition, had come back to life. The beaches were open. The parks were full of people. Restaurants had spread onto the sidewalks. The government had allowed professional sports to restart—without fans—and said that schools would reopen in the fall. New Yorkers were doing what they always did in the summer: barbecuing, exercising, partying, swimming. And shooting one another.

Shootings doubled in 2020 to a fourteen-year high. Murders rose 40 percent. Some people blamed the violence on bail reforms that had allowed defendants to remain free pending trial. Others said police were treading lightly because of the protests. Those were not views that I shared. In EMS, we saw what people were going through. They were under a lot of stress. They had been cooped up in small apartments or shelters since the spring. They had lost family members. They had lost their jobs. The city was boiling with anger and grief. And now I was in a nice house in Canarsie with one of the victims of those shootings.

An EMT knelt on the floor next to the patient. She had pushed aside the glass coffee table and was trying to examine his torso. A cop stood near his head. They each questioned him.

"Sir, do you have any preexisting medical conditions?" the EMT asked.

"No, I don't."

"Do you know the identity of the person or persons who shot you?" the cop asked.

"No."

"Sir, are you currently taking any medication?"

"No."

"How many shooters were there?"

"I don't remember."

The guy looked from the EMT to the cop and back, like someone watching a game of Ping-Pong. With the EMT, he was polite. With the cop, not so much.

"You gotta be able to remember how many shooters there were," the cop said. "One? Two?"

The patient's voice rose: "Listen, Officer. Some guys shot me and I'm trying to get some help here."

"Sir, do you know how many times you were shot?" the EMT asked, carefully lifting the man's T-shirt.

"I think they hit me once."

"What did they look like?" the cop asked.

"I don't know."

The cop wasn't buying it. I wasn't either. If "some guys" walk into your house and shoot you, you're going to remember something about them. Maybe that one was white, skinny, with a goatee, maybe that another was Black and wore a baseball cap. This guy claimed to know nothing, which told me that he knew a lot. Most likely, he knew exactly who'd shot him and why. Although he clearly had no intention of sharing that information with the cop.

Instead, he started yelling. "Don't take me to Brookdale," he wailed. "I don't want to go to Brookdale."

Brookdale University Hospital was the closest medical center. It was the logical destination for our patient. The hospital serves some of Brooklyn's poorest communities: Brownsville, East New York, East Flatbush. But for whatever reason, he didn't want to go there. Maybe he knew that somebody there would recognize him.

I knelt between the EMT and the cop. "Hey," I said. "Look at me. I need to talk to you. Was it a big gun or a small gun?" I asked. It makes a difference. Small-caliber bullets are more likely to ricochet off your bones and damage your insides. Big bullets just blast straight through.

"It was small," he said.

Out with the Raptor shears. We cut off the guy's shirt, cleaned the area around the wound, and applied a pressure dressing—a wad of gauze held in place with surgical tape—to stem the bleeding. As we worked on him, his mother walked in. She had short hair, graying a little at the temples. She was neatly dressed. She looked like she had come from work.

A typical mother would get pretty agitated if she came home from the office and found her son bleeding on the sofa and surrounded by police. This woman was very polite.

"Is he going to be okay?" she asked me quietly. "Did the bullet go through him?"

"No," I said, "the bullet's still inside him. He may need surgery to remove it." I added, "But he'll be fine. Don't worry."

I had palpated the patient's stomach, and it was soft. When there's internal bleeding, the cavity becomes full and rigid. So that was a good sign. His skin color was normal, not the ashen color of someone who has lost a lot of blood. I wasn't particularly worried about him.

We rolled the guy out to the ambulance. I jumped in the back with him and hooked him up to oxygen. (A patient who has lost blood has a diminished number of red blood cells, so we need to make sure that the ones that remain are carrying as much oxygen as possible.) We immobilized his neck just in case the bullet had injured his spine, although that seemed unlikely given where the wound was. Even though the bullet could have ricocheted, there weren't many bones in the lower abdomen for it to have bounced off.

A cop would travel with the patient to the hospital and probably cuff him there due to the suspicious circumstances in which he was shot. For now, though, that cop was waiting on the sidewalk, looking at his phone, while the other police officers went in and out of the house. It was just me, the patient, and, in the front of the ambulance, the EMT who was driving.

Suddenly, the patient tapped me on the arm. "Sir," he said.

"What's up?"

"I have something in the house."

"Like what?"

"A kilo of cocaine."

"Oh."

The EMT in the front seat turned to look at me. We both raised our eyebrows.

"Did the cops find it?" the man asked.

"I don't know," I said. I shrugged. "I think we would have heard by now if they had."

So now I was playing the priest as the guy from Canarsie made his confession. The ambulance has that effect on people. The patient is shut in a box with a paramedic or an EMT, seeing his life recede through the back doors of the ambulance. Let's say the patient overdosed. Or was shot. Or stabbed. That's the point when people realize that the choices they've made have consequences. So they start talking. They tell us things that they wouldn't share with their families. Especially not with their mothers.

"A kilo?" I asked the patient.

"Yeah."

A kilo of cocaine would fetch tens of thousands of dollars on the street. More important, a kilo of cocaine could land my patient in jail for a very long time.

"Please," he said. "Don't tell my mom."

I said nothing.

"I don't want my mom to know."

I nodded. What was it about men and their mothers? Here was a guy who had been shot by two or more violent individuals. They knew where he lived. He was about to be handcuffed and accompanied to the hospital by a member of the NYPD. There was yellow police tape across his front door. There were police milling around his home. If they found the quantity of cocaine he was talking about, he would face years in a dangerous penitentiary, the kind of place where Richie did time. His best option was probably to cooperate and give the cops information on the shooters. Which would mean trouble for him down the road.

But that was not what was worrying him. What was worrying him was the possibility that his mom might find out that he was dealing hard drugs. That the nice lady with the graying temples would discover the truth about her son.

I wouldn't volunteer the information to the cops, but I wouldn't lie to them if they asked. His mother, though—if she didn't know, I wasn't going to be the one to tell her.

"Don't worry," I said. "I won't tell your mom."

The guy in Canarsie reminded me of Richie. When I was thirteen years old, Richie lived for a time in a separate apartment on the top floor of the house in Park Slope. My parents let him stay there for free. He was twenty-six. He was home from Elmira.

I went up to the apartment one day to see him. Richie was in the bathroom. There was a guy sprawled on the couch. I recognized him, but I didn't know his name. He wore a New York Jets jacket, Irish green. He looked into the middle distance. He didn't say anything.

On the black coffee table in the living room, there were two triple beam scales, the kind we used in science class. Next to them were several bags of white powder. And a .38-caliber revolver. I didn't make the connection between the scales, the powder, and the gun. I just remember being surprised that Richie was into science like me.

Richie walked in. He saw me, the stash on the table, and the weapon, and he freaked out.

"Don't tell Mom," Richie said. Either he was scared of her or he didn't want to disappoint her—or both.

Mom worried about Richie all the time. Richie was in a fight; Richie was getting high; Richie was in jail. Richie had always had trouble keeping up at school—some kind of learning disability. It made Mom extremely protective. When Richie got into an argument with Johnny MG and knocked over his motorbike, it was Mom who waded into the fight and came out with two black eyes. When Richie cheated on his wife, Holly, Mom leaped to Richie's defense.

"You drove him to do that," Mom told Holly. "Don't come crying to me."

Mom was Richie's ally. He wasn't about to lose that.

"Promise me you won't tell Mom," Richie said again.

"Okay," I said. "I get it. I won't tell Mom."

There was another call, years ago, that made me think of Richie. When I was working at Station 38 with Joe, I picked up a shooting victim on Linden Boulevard in Crown Heights. The guy had just been to church. He'd been shot in the chest and the abdomen. The man's girlfriend screamed that the shooter was her ex-boyfriend.

We got the patient on the stretcher and rolled him into the back of the ambulance. He was bleeding heavily; blood was seeping through the four-by-four gauze bandages. He was African-American, but his skin was ashen. I couldn't get a blood pressure reading. The guy asked if I would hold his hand. I took it.

"Am I going to die?" he said.

I gulped. I knew I wasn't supposed to tell him the truth. The company line is to give patients hope, to tell them that they're going to be okay. But I felt this man wanted me to be straight with him.

I nodded quickly. "Yes, I think so," I said. "Is there anything that you want me to do?" I asked. "What do you need me to do for you?"

"Tell my daughter I love her very much," the man said. "And tell my mother that I'm sorry."

The guy didn't make it. I waited at the hospital for the man's mother. When she got there, at one a.m., I sat with her and delivered the message.

I'm sorry, Mom. I'm sorry. I sometimes wonder if those were the words that went through Richie's mind when Strike held the gun to his temple: *I'm sorry I let you down, Mom. I'm sorry I'm leaving you.*

Did Richie know that his death would destroy her? That it would ruin us all?

Sometimes patients want the truth but we have to keep it from them. One evening, a week or so after the call in Canarsie, Angie called me. She'd been at work. She sounded torn up.

"I had a COVID patient today, Anthony," she said. "It was so sad. I came home and cried my eyes out."

That didn't sound like Angie. During the pandemic, Angie didn't share a lot about the calls that she went on. Whenever I asked her how she was doing, she would say she was doing okay. That she was putting her feelings away and that she'd deal with them when everything got better. But since Matt died, Angie had been a little more fragile.

Angie had responded to a call in Bensonhurst. The man was in his seventies. He was in terrible shape. He had every underlying condition under the sun: heart disease, diabetes, high blood pressure, renal failure. His body was a creaky boat just waiting for COVID to sink it.

Angie checked the patient's oxygen saturation level. It was 68 percent, as low as Angie had seen on any patient during the pandemic. She knelt beside the man and put her gloved hand on his arm. "Sir, I'm going to have to intubate you," Angie said gently. "You're not getting enough oxygen by yourself. We need to give you oxygen. We're going to breathe for you."

The man looked stricken. "No," he gasped. "Please. I don't want that."

"I'm sorry," said Angie. "It's the only thing we can do. We have to help you breathe."

She grabbed an unopened IV bag and drip set and prepared to insert the IV. She tied a band around the patient's arm and pressed the inside of his elbow gently with her forefingers to locate the vein. She cleaned the site with an alcohol wipe. "Okay, you're going to feel a scratch," she said.

"I know I'm dying," the man said. His eyes searched Angie's face. He said, "I'm dying, and you don't want to tell me."

"Don't worry," Angie told him. "We're going to take care of you." But Angie could see this man was unlikely to live. He gurgled as he breathed, and his skin had a bluish tinge that indicated hypoxia.

"I'm not going to make it," the patient insisted. "I know I'm not."

"You're not going to die," Angie said. It pained her to lie to this man. She was about to sedate him and intubate him. When he got to the hospital he'd be put on a ventilator, and chances were he'd never wake up.

A few days after Angie transported the patient, she returned to the hospital. She asked about him and they told her that the man had died. If she'd told him the truth, Angie wondered, would it have helped him in some way? She'd never know. And it broke her heart.

At work, I was coiled like a spring. Ready to tear into somebody. Not any of the EMTs or paramedics—we had developed a real bond. We were the grunts who fought next to each other while the generals sat behind the lines. But I'd had it with the higher-ups: The voices on the other end of the phone who wanted me to time units when they came in for a bathroom break because they thought that the crews were slacking. The FDNY EMS operations office that sent buck slips informing us of yet more changes to our protocols. They were all so detached from what was going on in people's homes and on our ambulances that it made me fume.

Normally, I'm pretty civil at work, and I respect the hierarchy. I chew the department out on Twitter, but I'm a good soldier. After the spring of 2020, though, there were days when I lost it with people.

Like the day in mid-August that I was working overtime in Washington Heights, in upper Manhattan, well outside of my usual zone. I walked into the apartment of a Dominican family to find five or six people sitting around the bed of a very elderly woman. The grandmother, I assumed. The woman was motionless.

I stood in the doorway. A paramedic crew had arrived before I did. One of the family—a guy in his forties—stood up.

"It's my mother," he said. "She passed away."

He said the woman had breathed her last an hour earlier. The family had tied a little scarf around her face to prevent her jaw from dropping open.

One of the medics was in the hallway outside the bedroom speaking to telemetry. I heard her explaining the situation. The patient had stopped breathing an hour ago, she said. There was no lividity yet. No rigor mortis.

"So, you want me to give her an amp of epi and an amp of bicarb and work her up?" the medic said. She sounded skeptical.

I looked at the woman lying peacefully on the bed. There was no way that I was going to have the paramedics drag her from the bed to the floor and start cracking her frail ribs.

"Here, give me the phone," I said to the medic. She passed it to me. "Doc, this is Lieutenant Almojera. The family does not want us to work the patient up."

"You have to work her up," the doctor said.

I knew the doctor. This was his boilerplate response.

"Give the patient an amp of epi and bicarb and intubate," he said in a flat voice.

The doctor wanted the medics to put an IV in the woman's limp arm and inject her lifeless veins with epinephrine and sodium bicarbonate. To remove the scarf that her family had thoughtfully tied around her face so they could tip back her head, force a laryngoscope blade into her throat, and stick a tube inside of her. All while vigorously pumping her chest. As her family watched.

The patient appeared to have died of old age. She had died at home, with her family around her. She had been granted the peaceful death that was denied to so many COVID victims, all those patients who'd had to die while their relatives watched on iPads. And now, a doctor in an office in Queens wanted us to desecrate her body just to follow the rules on a piece of paper.

No way.

"I'd like you to give me a time of death," I said.

"You know the protocols, Lieutenant."

Yes, the protocols. Those had changed again. The department had lifted the twenty-minute rule for CPR, so we were back to our non-COVID regulations. There was no longer a time limit on efforts to resuscitate a patient. This was a positive thing. It was what we were used to. But it was hard to snap back to the old ways. One week, lieutenants were telling medics and EMTs to limit care and stop CPR after twenty minutes if there was no pulse. The next week, they were telling them to keep their efforts up for as long as they thought necessary, to try to revive everyone. Even an old lady who had quietly slipped away in her bed.

"Wait, Doc. Two months ago, the department said I had to stop CPR on a thirty-five-year-old COVID patient who was otherwise healthy and whose family was begging us to do more because his twenty minutes was up, and we didn't have enough hands to cope with the pandemic. And now you want me to work up a ninety-one-year-old woman who has been dead for an hour against her family's wishes?

"Doc, I want a time of death," I said.

"You know what the rules are," the doctor said.

"I do," I said. "And I know how you change them to suit the situation."

Throughout the spring, we'd been forced to make hard decisions because the medical system was collapsing, forced to ration care and explain to families that we couldn't take their loved ones to the hospital. With the old lady who'd died in bed, we had a chance to restore the humanity to our work. Instead of following the rules blindly, we could make a choice that would allow her some dignity in death.

"I want a time of death, Doc."

There was a pause. Then the doctor said, "Sixteen fifty-eight."

"Sixteen fifty-eight?" I repeated.

"Yes," he said coldly. "Sixteen fifty-eight."

We pronounced the woman dead. Her son stood up and shook my hand.

SEPTEMBER 2020

On a cool morning in late September, I sat on a wooden piling that stuck out of the sand on Coney Island beach. The day was fresh and clear, just like the day a year earlier when I'd bumped into Joe at Villabate Alba, the Italian pastry joint. I was working overtime. It was around seven a.m. and the Dispatch radio was quiet, so I'd driven to the eastern end of Coney Island, parked near the beach, and walked out onto the sand.

I had just scheduled the surgery to repair my torn biceps tendon. Hospitals and clinics were back to doing nonurgent procedures. My original surgeon had caught COVID and was convalescing, so I'd had to find a new one. But now it was settled: October 29 at an outpatient surgery center in Gramercy Park. I'd be off work for three months and spend another three months on light duty—deskbound, in other words.

I was glad to have a date, but I was apprehensive. About the operation, the recovery. Being stuck at home alone.

I was also anxious about money. I'd receive full pay from the fire department while I was recovering, but full pay without overtime—and without the income from my extra gigs at Aqueduct and at the defibrillator company—amounted to half of what I normally earned. And the only reason that I would be paid at all was that my injury counted as line-of-duty. If I'd done this to myself outside of work, I would have had to use sick days and vacation days to cover my time off. And when I ran out of leave, I'd have been taken off payroll. And once I was off payroll for a month, I'd have lost my health insurance.

And what is a line-of-duty injury, anyway? If a paramedic who has carted two-hundred-fifty-pound patients on a stair chair for two decades throws out her back bending to pick up her house keys, is the injury connected to her work? I think so. Many Americans punish their bodies day in and day out cleaning floors and processing meat and running around sweltering warehouses. And when they become sick or injured, what kind of health-care coverage do they have? At least my injury had happened on the job. And I had insurance.

With my surgery on the horizon, I started wading through mounds of paperwork related to disability pay and insurance. And to save some money, I worked overtime wherever I could get it.

Which, on that September morning, was in one of my favorite spots. I love working near the ocean—Coney Island, the Rockaways in Queens. Life in the beach communities is different. People seem to live more slowly. They walk and bike and fish.

There are a few FDNY EMS units that patrol the New York beaches in Gators, which are souped-up golf carts with stretchers on the back. Those EMTs have tans and sunglasses—a little like those *Baywatch* medics that Angie and I chatted with in Sydney. They're the envy of all EMS workers. Sadly, there are no Gator-riding lieutenant paramedics. Oceanside overtime was my consolation.

The morning was quiet. A group of Chinese men fished from the pier, where there are plenty of flounder. A man in his seventies power-walked along the wet sand beside the water. He was shirtless and wore a white golf cap. A gold chain hanging in his chest hair caught the sunlight.

I glanced back at the boardwalk. A couple of cyclists rode toward Brighton Beach. The boardwalk at Coney Island is nearly three miles long. It's clean and well kept. It wasn't like that when I was a kid. Back then, there were people living underneath it. I'd look down through the broken boards and see pairs of eyes staring up at me.

I listened to the BBC on my AirPods. The number of cases of COVID was rising around the world, and a quarter of a million people were testing positive each day. European countries that had opened their doors to tourists in the summer were locking down again because of a spike in infections.

In the United States, the coronavirus situation didn't seem to be getting worse, at least. Nationwide, the number of new cases each day had dropped from about sixty-six thousand in July to forty thousand in mid-September. Around seven hundred people were dying daily.

And in New York, the virus was still quiet. There were days in September when five people or fewer died from the virus. Five. Compared to over nine hundred people dying on some days in the spring.

But in EMS, we knew that we weren't shot of the virus. Experts predicted an increase in infections in the fall. It made sense; seasonal viruses spread better in cold weather, and they thrive in schools, which had been open—for some students, anyway—for a week or so.

The idea of going back into a storm of COVID like the one we had been through in spring was unbearable. Yes, we had the experience of the spring to guide us. But I didn't know a soul in EMS who felt mentally sturdy enough to endure another surge in infections and deaths.

My circle of friends had been wobbly since Matt Keene's death. Angie was a little more somber, as if Matt's death had brought her sadness closer to the surface. Mike was also very upset. And Andres wasn't the same person he'd been before he found Matt's body. Who would be? Every time somebody mentioned Matt, he fell quiet.

I thought about Joe. It had been nearly a year since he'd died. I wondered what he would have made of the pandemic. He would have been pissed about the lack of support from the fire department, that's for sure. But Joe hadn't even heard of SARS-CoV-2. Maybe that was a good thing. He was spared having to witness all this suffering.

I took off my shoes and socks and walked down to the edge of the water. Strictly speaking, I shouldn't stray that far from the command vehicle, even when it's parked. I definitely shouldn't be barefoot. But it felt good to turn my back on the craziness of the city—the pandemic, the shootings, the stabbings, the nonsense—and stare at the empty expanse of water. It was comforting to think that all the fish and crustaceans below the waves had no idea that a virus had brought humanity to a tragic standstill. They were just down there swimming and hiding under rocks, I thought. Eating each other and going about their lives.

I'd barely been to the beach all summer, and now the summer was ending. During a normal summer, I went a few times a month. I'd get there very early, bring a chair and a Bluetooth speaker. Buy a nutcracker—a lethal (and illicit) rum and vodka cocktail in a small plastic bottle—from the guys who hawk them on the beach. But going to the beach during the summer of 2020 felt very constrained. You had to wear a mask and keep your distance, even in the sea.

I stepped into the shallow water. It was as still as a pond. The waves lapped softly against the sand. I rolled up the pants of my uniform to just above my calves. I wiggled my toes. The sea tugged the sand from beneath them. I felt as if I were floating.

I stood there for ten minutes or so. Then I walked back to the wooden piling where I'd left my shoes and sat there while my feet dried. I wanted to savor the moment. I felt more peaceful than I had in weeks.

The radio broke my reverie. "Four-Three Charlie, take it over to Brighton Sixth Street and the boardwalk for the drowning."

"Four-Three Charlie. Show us sixty-three."

I grabbed my shoes, shoved my feet into them. No socks.

I ran up the beach.

The victim had been swimming in the sea off Brighton Beach, about a mile east of the spot where I was sitting. She was in her early fifties. Moderate build. Not especially fit. She wore a navy one-piece swimsuit, and her toenails were painted pink. There was a crowd of people around her: Firefighters in wet suits. Cops in wet suits. Swimmers. By-standers. A blue and white NYPD boat sat in the water about ten yards from the shore.

An EMT crew—Four-Three Charlie—was working on the woman. One of the EMTs pumped her chest.

"What happened?" I asked.

"Guy saw her struggling in the water. Called 911," one of the fire-fighters said. He nodded toward a man in his forties who was looking on. "Cop boat picked her up."

When the police found the woman, she wasn't breathing, the fire-fighter said. The police boat had brought her close to the shore, and the firefighters had lifted her off and carried her through the water onto the sand.

"I figure she had an MI in the water," one of the paramedics said. A myocardial infarction. That made sense. It seemed unlikely that she'd had trouble swimming—the water was calm and the tide was not pulling hard.

The medic grabbed a towel and briskly dried the woman off, since we couldn't shock her while she was wet. The medic placed electrode pads on the patient's chest. The monitor showed ventricular fibril-lation, meaning her heart was quivering like the heart of the truck driver Daniel who we'd saved on the bridge the previous winter. The paramedics shocked her. Resumed CPR. Checked the monitor.

Now there was no electrical activity at all. The patient's heart was flatline.

The medics inserted an IV and gave the woman an amp of epi.

Still nothing.

"Let's get her off the beach," I said. "You gonna intubate?"

We would have to drag the woman over the sand in the sked, a flexible device shaped like a taco that we use when we can't roll a stretcher. It would be hard to pump air into her lungs using a bag-valve mask while we transported her. There would be too much movement. The best bet was to intubate now, before we started moving. That way, we'd have a definitive airway as we dragged the sked.

The medics intubated the patient while the EMTs continued CPR.

"Listen up," I said. We wouldn't be able to move the patient and do CPR at the same time, so we would have to drag her, stop and do a round of CPR, then drag her again. We'd alternate moving her and pumping her chest until we reached the ambulance.

"We're gonna move for thirty seconds and stop, do CPR for two minutes, then carry." Each time we stopped, a different EMT or firefighter would take over CPR, then step aside while we moved the patient. We call it CPR in transit. The crews knew the drill.

They cocooned the patient in the sked. "Are we ready to roll?" I asked. "Here we go."

We dragged the sked a short distance over the sand. One of the firefighters timed it. "Thirty seconds," he said.

"Stop," I said. "Compressions."

We huddled around the sked. One of the team members compressed the woman's chest while the firefighter kept track of the time.

"Two minutes."

The medic checked the monitor. "Still asystole," she said. "Another amp of epi going in."

It took close to ten minutes to get the patient from the water to the boardwalk. A crew waited there with a stretcher.

We got the patient onto the stretcher and continued CPR. The medics called telemetry. They were given the order to administer sodium bicarbonate and calcium chloride—the medications we turn to in the field when epinephrine isn't enough to restart a person's heart.

Then they loaded the patient and drove away. I climbed into my truck and followed the ambulance. They were heading to Coney Island Hospital.

The medics kept up CPR all the way, but there was no change. In the emergency department, the doctor pronounced the woman dead.

Afterward, I stood in the ambulance bay with the medics. They were covered in sand.

"That was quite a workout," one said.

"You all did great," I told them.

"Thanks, Lou," one of the medics said. "It's a shame we couldn't save her."

"Take your time. Clean up. Sand is a bitch to get rid of."

I thought about the woman going out that morning for her swim. And about the fact that, while she drowned, I was standing with my feet in the same water.

As I walked back to my truck, I could feel the sand between my toes.

A week or so earlier, I'd had my first session of eye movement desensitization and reprocessing—a psychotherapy method that helps people process trauma. Like so much else in 2020, the counseling session took place on Zoom. I sat at the table in my kitchen. It was a warm evening, so I wore a T-shirt and shorts.

The therapist was middle-aged. She was calling from what looked like her living room. She explained the process of EMDR, which involves breathing and visualization. The therapist gets you to think of a traumatic memory while you're watching your fingers move from side to side or while tapping yourself in a rhythmic way.

I had received a call in July from the NYC Trauma Recovery Network, an organization that offers pro bono EMDR therapy. The NYC TRN was created after the World Trade Center attacks to help first responders, survivors, and family members. Now the group was offering sessions to members of the FDNY EMS corps. The coronavirus pandemic was our 9/11, after all. Someone from the network had seen me on television talking about the psychological toll of the pandemic on EMS and contacted me to set up the free therapy sessions. At least all the media interviews I was doing were having an impact, I thought.

The TRN said it could offer six to ten free sessions of EMDR to any EMS member who wanted it. The EMS FDNY Help Fund—a nonprofit that supports EMTs and medics who are facing hardship—said it would chip in for additional sessions if somebody needed them.

Around the time that TRN called me, I reached out to the National Institute for the Psychotherapies to set up long-term therapy for EMS members outside the department. With the NIP in the mix, members would have a choice of different therapeutic approaches—talk therapy, which is long term, and EMDR, which is short term.

EMS members were frustrated with the way the FDNY Counseling Service Unit was handling things. I have used the CSU. The counselors are good, and they do their best. But the unit was set up to deal with the trauma of 9/11, when hundreds of firefighters were killed in a single day. It wasn't set up to deal with emergency medical service workers coping with a pandemic. The unit had limited hours and few locations where you could see a counselor.

When the EMDR therapist described the method to me, I was a little doubtful. I've been in therapy on and off for seventeen years, and sometimes I feel like I've tried everything. Like I'm talked out. Like I've raked over my past and learned how to avoid repeating mistakes, but then I repeat them anyway.

I was willing to give EMDR a try, though. For one thing, I was hoping to encourage other EMS members to do it. By taking the TRN up on its offer of sessions, I could set an example.

And I was curious about the method. It was more targeted than talk therapy. It would teach me techniques to get through moments of anger or fear or panic. And, ideally, it would help me reprogram my brain to find traumatic memories less painful.

"Okay, Anthony," the therapist said. "Let's talk about what's going on with you. What's upsetting you?"

"Anger," I said. "Not sleeping. Stress."

I talked about how I was lucky if I slept four hours a night. How I woke up in the wee hours. How not sleeping fed my frustration and sense of defeat because I knew I was going to be exhausted before I even started my day.

"Take your index and middle finger. Tap them on your forehead in a rhythm. One, two. One, two. Count the taps. As you tap, think about the thing that's making you angry. Picture the anger or the thing that's bothering you. Tap. Give me something that's bothering you, Anthony," she said. "Give me something you're afraid of."

Tap-tap, tap-tap, tap-tap.

I thought about the woman I had been dating who was now dating somebody else.

"Now tap your cheeks," the therapist said.

I thought about my parents. About how my mother literally pushed me out into the world and then, for most part, left me to figure things out by myself. About how Mom and Dad took it for granted that I could look after myself. About how they weren't here now, when I needed their support.

"Now move your hands down and tap your chin."

I thought about the fire department, the endless fights to get workers what they deserved. About the injustice of the pandemic and how the most vulnerable communities had suffered its consequences.

I thought of Joe and Greg and Tony Thomas.

Of Little Eddie. Donna and Mimi.

Of Chris and Anthony.

Of Richie.

The whole session, I tapped. I learned tapping techniques to help me sleep. Tapping that would calm me down.

At the end, I didn't feel all that different, but I'd enjoyed having a person to talk to for an hour, someone solely focused on me. Enjoyed being the cared for rather than the caregiver.

After the first session, I did another. I agreed to stay the course. For a while, I used the techniques. When I couldn't sleep, I tapped. I slept a little better.

But I quickly started slipping. I had a lot on my plate. I'd started taking college classes again so that I could finish my degree. I was working long hours. I didn't use the EMDR techniques consistently.

It wasn't the method that was the problem. It was me.

The fact was, I was spiraling into darkness. At work, I was sluggish. Unenthusiastic. A little snappish. On my days off, I stayed home. I lay on my couch and hugged a pillow. I streamed movies and scrolled through Twitter.

When I did socialize with friends, I felt as if there was a veil hanging between me and everyone else. I went out one night in September for Italian food with Angie, Jonathan, Sara, Dre, and one or two others. We talked. People laughed. But I felt as if I were hovering outside the group, looking at them through a foggy window. The conversation was a meaningless noise, like the *wa-wa-wa* of Charlie Brown's teacher in the *Peanuts* cartoons.

I didn't want to have to do the work. I didn't want to talk. I didn't want to tap. I didn't want to breathe and hold my posture. I wanted someone to snap his fingers and have everything go away. I was tired of trying to fix myself.

At the end of September, I found myself back in Brighton Beach, this time in a low-rise apartment building a couple of blocks from the sea.

The patient was an eighty-four-year-old man. He was Russian. He lived with his wife in a railroad apartment. Very clean and neat.

I arrived with a crew of paramedics. We were the first on scene. We went through the apartment to the bedroom.

The man was lying on a bed that had a cedar-colored headboard. There was a nightstand beside the bed. Very little other furniture.

He was gulping air like a fish. Agonal breathing. It's not real breathing; it's a reflex that happens when the brain is starved of oxygen, often due to cardiac arrest or stroke.

The patient didn't show signs of being sick with COVID. He wasn't sweating or feverish. But he was close to death.

His wife sat next to him on the bed. She was a stout woman in her late seventies. She wore a light blue smock with pockets. She leaned over her husband and patted his shoulder. She spoke to him softly in Russian.

It's okay, she seemed to be saying. *It's okay. It's okay.*

As we walked into the room, she looked up. She stood to let the medics pass. Then she walked out of the bedroom.

The paramedics pulled the man onto the floor so they could start CPR. They inserted an IV in the patient's arm and intubated him. They put electrodes on his chest to check his heart.

There was no electrical activity. The man had died.

I went into the living room. The paramedics would remove the IV and the breathing tube. They'd put the man back onto the bed and pull up the sheets.

His wife was sitting on the edge of a couch covered in plastic. She leaned on the arm of the couch and looked out of the window at the street.

I wondered if she and her husband had come to this country together, wondered how many decades they had been married. What kind of life they had built together.

I approached her. She looked up. I removed my gloves. I bent and put my hand on her shoulder. We'd come a long way from the day in Sheepshead Bay when I'd had to stand several feet from that inconsolable man. The infection rates now were low enough that we could drop our guard a little.

"I'm afraid he's gone," I said. "There's nothing more that we can do for him."

The woman looked into my face. Her eyes were blue, like her smock. Her expression was soft. She didn't look surprised or disbelieving. It was as if she accepted her husband's death.

She put her hand on top of mine and slowly patted it, like a grandmother soothing a child.

"It's okay," she said in English. "It's okay."

A few minutes later, the police arrived. They would take custody of the body. The medics and I gathered our equipment. I asked the woman if she wanted to be with her husband. She nodded. She went into the room and sat next to him on the bed.

As we left, she was stroking his hair.

Epilogue

The room was dark. Light from a streetlamp shone through the window next to the bed. I'm often up before dawn, so I rarely close the blinds. Outside, the street was quiet. Muffled with snow.

I picked up my phone to check the time, hoping it would be around five or six. That it would be close to dawn and the world would soon be stirring. But it was two in the morning.

I sighed. Closed my eyes again. Tried to still my brain.

I breathed. Slowly in, slowly out.

Thoughts floated through my mind like the phosphenes making squiggles inside my eyelids. A fight with an EMS chief over whether ambulances could sit at the station during the snowstorm. The Orthodox Jewish family who lived across the street from me. Was anyone awake in that house? I wondered. Was anyone lying in bed worrying?

In the distance, a car engine hummed, then stopped. A door slammed. The car started up again. My body began to feel heavy, relaxed. I drifted off.

Then my leg jerked. I felt a flutter of adrenaline. My mind crackled to life.

Shit.

I was wide awake.

. . .

It was early February 2021. A blizzard had smothered the city on the first of the month, the day I returned to work after three months' leave. The snow cheered me up a little. Sure, blizzards are a pain. Our ambulances get stuck in the drifts that clog New York's streets, and we have to lift patients over the banks of snow created by the plows. But I like the change of rhythm. And the city loses its sharp edges. It becomes romantic. Even our sirens don't sound so piercing.

I'd had surgery on my biceps tendon at the end of October, just over a year after I'd torn it while trying to catch Joe on his stretcher. Outpatient procedure. It had gone well. Angie, Kala, and Sara had driven me to the clinic in Manhattan and waited six hours so they could bring me home. Terence had swung by while I was in the recovery room.

The surgeon had made a crosswise incision just below the inside of my left elbow. He'd drilled a hole in the radius, one of the bones in the forearm. He'd stitched a tiny metal button to the part of the tendon that was still attached to my biceps, then he'd threaded the tendon through the hole and anchored it on the other side using the button.

Just before the surgery team put me under, I'd made a joke about the Manchester United tattoo on the back of my left forearm. I hoped there were no Liverpool supporters on the team, I said. I wouldn't want them to tank the procedure on purpose.

When I came to, the doctor told me that the tendon had been rubbery enough to stretch through the bone. He hadn't needed to take one from a corpse. This meant I'd heal more easily and recover most of my strength. The surgeon couldn't remember the last time he'd been able to save a tendon that had been retracted for so many months. For the first time in ages, it seemed, I had gotten lucky.

Spending three months at home was everything I'd feared it would be. Boring, isolating. I should have been relieved to have time off, especially after the year that we'd had in EMS. But my friends work long hours, so I was by myself a lot of the time. It was lonely.

Not that I was short of help or company. Friends visited. For a month after my surgery, I wore a soft cast that was bent at the elbow with an L-shaped metal shank to prevent me from straightening my arm. I had to thread a plastic bag over it when I took a shower. Before I mastered the art of doing this, I asked an ex-girlfriend to come over and help me. She was an EMT. She was the only person I could undress in front of without feeling too self-conscious.

And I received help from unexpected quarters. About three weeks after my surgery, I went hiking in Westchester with Mike. I took the 2 train to meet him, and he drove the rest of the way. I couldn't tie my shoelaces, so before I got on the subway, I approached some kids smoking weed near the entrance.

"Brothers, can you help me?" I said. "I'm in a bit of a jam."

One of the kids knelt down and tied my shoes. I offered him some money. He wouldn't take it. It was a small gesture, but it made my day.

As we hiked, I talked to Mike about how I was having a hard time letting go of my last relationship. It bothered me that my ex had never sat me down and said, *It's over, and this is why.* That she didn't have the guts to tell me she didn't want me.

That had been happening all my life. My parents never acknowledged that they'd dropped the ball, that they'd gone on with their lives and damaged mine in the process. Even when my dad was dying of liver failure, he didn't want to talk about anything. The same thing happened with women. They drifted off or cheated on me; they rarely made a clean break.

"The thing about these women, Ant, is that you're attracted to fixer-uppers. Women who you think you can help," Mike said. "But those women aren't looking for a guy who's sensitive and vulnerable. They're probably looking for a guy with swagger and money to burn. Someone to distract them."

"I don't pick them, Mike. They pick me," I said. "And then I see they need help. So I help. But as soon as they bounce back, they're gone."

"That's the thing, though, Anthony. They don't ask for your help. You volunteer it. And the same shit happens every time."

"Wait. I show empathy and patience with a woman," I said, "I help her through tough times, then the moment I show some vulnerability, she leaves me. How is that my fault?" I knew Mike was right. I just wasn't in the mood to listen.

"Look, Anthony," Mike said. "The way I see this is that the universe is protecting you. These are not the women you want to be having a relationship with. They don't deserve you."

Mike said he'd lie down in front of my car if necessary to prevent me from seeing a woman like that again. He was kidding, but only kind of. And for a moment, he made me feel better.

From the sidelines, I was able to do a little something to fight the virus. In December, I got my first shot of the vaccine. The FDA had given emergency approval for the vaccines made by Pfizer-BioNTech and Moderna. I got the Moderna shot, with a follow-up dose in January.

The debate over the vaccine drove me nuts. It was a replay of the nonsense over masks. People didn't trust the science. They didn't see why they should do something to protect themselves or their community. Even in the fire department, only a third of firefighters and EMS workers had signed up to get it. Some were afraid it would harm them. Some thought it was all part of a big conspiracy.

I wanted to encourage union members to get vaccinated, so I wore my union jacket and had the FDNY cameras photograph me getting the shot. We were in the middle of a post-Thanksgiving COVID surge. More than three thousand people a day were dying in the United States. And we were letting ideology get in the way of our health. Again. It's not like I thought that getting jabbed for the cameras would change much. But I wanted to do something.

I tried to keep myself distracted while I waited to go back to work. I organized a trip to Niagara Falls for New Year's Eve with Terence,

Vanessa, Angie, and Jonathan, her boyfriend. A couple of other friends. It took nine hours to get there on the train. We drank champagne and went to the casino. It was fun. But I was very aware of being on my own. After we counted down to the New Year, Angie kissed Jonathan; Terence and Vanessa kissed. It was hard to believe that a year earlier, I'd been watching fireworks in Sydney Harbor with no idea of what was to come.

In January, I took two classes, Russian and art. I was finishing up my degree at Brooklyn College, on track to graduate in June. My college diploma was twenty years in the making, but I'd be the first Almojera to get one.

Art class was a revelation. I bought canvases, brushes, acrylic paints, oil paints. I painted a still life of the potted plant that I'd bought when I joined the fire department. I spent nine straight hours on an oil painting of a woman walking down a rainy street. I sketched the woman dozens of times before she looked right. It was frustrating, but in the end, the painting looked how I wanted it to look.

If you took an EKG of my mood during January, it would have looked like a sinus bradycardia—a normal but very slow heartbeat. A line interrupted by occasional bumps. Except that if the bumps were as rare as mine were, the person would be dead. There were things that I found satisfying or fun, like painting, cooking a meal, taking a trip with friends. But the diversion was fleeting. In the space between activities, the joylessness returned.

Everything was tinged with pessimism. When I shopped for groceries, I dwelled on the fact that I was shopping for one. If I passed a pretty house on the street, I thought about how I'd probably never own property in this city and the likelihood that the family living in that house was unhappy.

It was self-indulgent. It was as if my misery had its own gravity that sucked the world in. But I couldn't help it.

Going back to work in late January lifted my mood a little. It was nice to catch up with my coworkers, to have company. But the heaviness soon returned. I was living on Jupiter. The simplest things took two and a half times the energy that they should have.

Now, a week after returning to work, I lay in bed and stared into the darkness.

My eyes felt scratchy. I had a slight headache. I noticed my heartbeat. My breathing. I could feel the blood rushing through the vessels in my brain. I became aware of all the work my organs were doing just to keep me alive.

Such an effort, I thought.

My mind buzzed from one outrage to the next like an angry insect. The insurrection at the Capitol a month earlier. The lies about the election. The cynicism of Republican politicians. The city officials who wanted to deny EMS workers a pay increase. After all that EMS had been through, after all the talk about what heroes first responders were, they wanted to stiff us.

Our society is so fucked up, I thought. We'd learned nothing. The spring had exposed the holes in our health-care system, but the city wasn't going to do a thing to mend them. All the talk of fighting inequality and social injustice was just talk—nothing more. New York had been hit by a metaphorical meteor in the spring, and we still had people who wouldn't wear a mask, who didn't want to get vaccinated.

During these dark nighttime rages, I felt like I was done with those people. If they died, they died.

All my life, I'd had faith in humanity. Not in politicians or family, but in the goodness of individual people. The guy with the blunt who had tied my shoes. The driver in India who, years later, had sent me a reclining Buddha in the mail.

Now, I thought, goodness had not won. It had lost to selfishness. Ignorance. Intolerance.

As I lay on my back, the bed felt as if it were expanding. Spreading toward the edges of the room. I turned onto my left side and stretched my arm across the mattress. Looked at my belly. I weighed two hundred and seventy-eight pounds. The price of my quest for comfort.

I closed my eyes. I felt like I was sinking, like water was closing over my head. In my mind, people swam past: Richie. Mom. Dad. I reached out. But they were made of water. I tried to swim to the surface. I gasped for breath.

I turned onto my back again. Tears trickled over my ears and onto the pillow.

Why do I have to do this? I thought. Why did I care so much about a city that didn't care about me? That didn't care for its people? Why did I want to fix EMS? Why couldn't I get other people to care as much as I did? I understood. They had families to worry about. They didn't have time to fight. They left it to Anthony. Because Anthony had the time, and Anthony needed someone to fight with.

You don't have to be this unhappy, Anthony. That's what people would say. *There are paths out.* But the paths were so steep. And I was so tired.

Fuck everyone, I thought. *I don't have the energy to do the work anymore. I don't have reasons.*

I don't know how long I lay in bed. But when I sat up, it was still dark.

Next to my bed, I had a green pocketknife. It was my travel knife. I'd been organizing my stuff the day before and I'd found it.

I picked up the knife and went into the bathroom. The bathroom is cream and yellow and a little drab. I opened the knife and put it on the edge of the tub. Then I climbed into the bath and sat with my knees bent.

Sometimes, when I am feeling detached from the world, I stand in the tub and turn the water on. I let it flow over me. The sensation of water running over my face, my chest, and my arms helps me reconnect with my body and with the world. But now, I didn't switch on the water. I leaned my head against the ledge behind me and closed my eyes.

If you work in EMS, visualizing a suicide is not an act of imagination. You've seen most of the ways that people choose to end their lives. The ones who jump. The ones who hang themselves. The ones who take pills. The ones who shoot themselves. The ones who cut their wrists.

You know it's something people do. And you get plenty of opportunities to contemplate how you'd do it.

Years earlier, I had resolved that if I ever decided to kill myself, I would wear underwear. I'd seen too many naked suicides. I wouldn't want to be found that way, especially not by people who knew me. If I didn't show up to work, the lieutenant closest to my house would be dispatched to check on me. If he or she couldn't get into the apartment, an engine company would be sent to force entry. Once they'd found me, they'd call in an EMT unit, to process the paperwork, and a police unit, to take custody. They'd all be crowded into my apartment: cops, firefighters, paramedics, the lieutenant. I wanted to be at least halfway presentable.

I'd also decided that I would keep it tidy. Somebody would have to clean up the scene, after all. A friend, a family member. I remember a call to a man who'd jumped off the overpass that crosses Fort Hamilton Parkway in Brooklyn. He was an Orthodox Jew. Orthodox people believe that anything that's in your body must be buried with you. So as we waited with the body, a group of women came and started mopping up the blood and remains of the patient from the asphalt with towels.

I knew that if you slashed your wrists, you should keep your hands inside the tub to contain the mess. And you should make the cut lengthwise. Not crosswise, the way people do it in films. If you cut across your wrist, you will most likely miss the artery. And the blood can clot, and the wound will stop bleeding. If you cut lengthwise, you can cut along the artery. That way, you make sure you bleed.

The Buddha teaches acceptance. Acceptance of the hardships of life, of loneliness, of the fact that life will end. It's stupid to cling to existence, because we'll continue to exist after this life as an essence of some sort. In nature documentaries, the prey tries to flee and then struggles in the cheetah's mouth. But eventually it goes limp. It acquiesces. Now, I thought, it was time to acquiesce.

I wouldn't write a note. I'd let them wonder. Let them stew. I pictured the women who had hurt me over the years. They would come to my funeral. They'd ask themselves if this was their fault. I imagined Angie at the funeral, kicking some of those women out. *You didn't love him enough when he was alive,* she'd say. *You can get the fuck out now.*

Then I pictured Angie at the moment that she learned that I was gone. Biting her lip. Trying not to cry. And then crying until her whole body shook.

I imagined Mike lifting his head to look skyward, the way he had when he heard about Matt Keene. But Mike is a million times closer to me than he was to Matt. He'd be destroyed. He'd already lost one brother. Now he'd have lost two.

And Mike and Angie would have to tell the rest of the Group Home. They'd have to tell Yvonne. Mike's the executor of my will, so it would fall to him to clear up the remnants of my life. He and Marshall would share my pension. A group of my friends would receive my life insurance.

But they'd have all that shit to sort out. And they'd be devastated. They wouldn't be the same afterward. I would be fucking with their lives.

Why would I do that to them? Why would I let my death dictate how my friends lived? Richie did that. Richie changed the course of my family's lives. Of everything. And even though Richie courted death, he didn't *know* he was going to die. What I'd be doing would be worse.

In 2009, on St. Patrick's Day, I was dispatched to a suicide on the Upper East Side of Manhattan. I'd been working the parade when the call came in. A middle-aged man had hung himself from the back of his bathroom door. He had lost a lot of money in the crash in 2008. He left a note for his wife asking her to call the police. *Don't enter the bathroom,* the note said. The man must have felt so much shame.

After we examined the body, I'd sat at the kitchen table with the man's wife. She held a tissue. Her eyes were red. She said she didn't understand why her husband had felt he couldn't share his burden.

"I would have gone through this with him," she told me. "He didn't have to think he was alone."

Angie, I thought.

Mike.

Dre. Jessa. Johana. Kala.

Manny. Marshall. Pete. Sara.

Terence. Wes. Zak.

A faint glow began to lighten the bathroom window. Out there were my friends, the family that I'd chosen. The people, broken in their ways, who still wanted to fix me. Who'd make sure that I was never alone.

Acknowledgments

This book is dedicated to the Group Home, who provide all the love and support a brother could need. Thank you, *mi famiglia:* Michael Sullivan, Marshall Johnson, Wes Tibbetts, Terence Lau, Peter Borriello, Andres Segovia Jr., Chris Marquart, Zak Mercer, Jose Gonzalez Jr., Manaury Reyes, and Mike Keegan; Angie Alburquerque, Sara Lupin, Kala Gabler, Jessa Tibbetts, Vanessa Kwan, Jenelle Pierre, Johana Clerge, Joanna Colon-Tellefson, Beth Marquart, Bibi Alladin, Liana Espinal, Nancy Khoury-Derosa, Ana Chaer, Korinna Litvinova, and Nicole Keegan. Family is bigger than the circle of people related to you by blood. You mean more to me than you will ever know.

A special thanks to my parents, who did the best they could with the tools they had. To my sister, Yvonne, who got the brunt of Richard and Linda and yet endured. You're one of the strongest people I know. To my brother, Richie, who never found peace in life. I learned the lessons, big brother, and I hope you found what you were looking for in the hereafter.

This book began, in a sense, with the actor Jeffrey Wright, who had the temerity to suggest I take part in a panel discussing the pandemic and its effects on society. Endless thanks to Jeffrey for his support in getting the word out about the tragedies and triumphs of EMS and to Jeffrey's foundation, Brooklyn for Life!, for feeding us.

Thank you also to Bryan Doerries and his Theater of War production team, in particular Marjolaine Goldsmith, for giving the EMS community—and me—a platform. Bryan's commitment to veterans and communities on the front lines is remarkable. And the way he helps us understand our vulnerabilities through Greek tragedy is truly unique.

A heartfelt thank you to Zoë Pagnamenta and her colleagues at the Zoë Pagnamenta Agency. Zoë saw me on Bryan's panel and believed I might have a story to tell. I am eternally grateful for her faith and guidance on the journey to this book.

Huge thanks, too, to Alex Littlefield and his team at HarperCollins and Mariner Books. They shepherded me through the editing and publishing process with wisdom, encouragement, and patience.

To Victoria Burnett, who took my thoughts and words and helped shape them into a story that the world would want to read. There are no words to convey the love and appreciation I have for you and all you have done to make this book happen. You are now an official member of the Group Home; in for a penny, in for a pound. Thank you, too, to Victoria's family—Paul, Olivia, and Max—for sharing her with me during this process.

A special thank you to Seema Reza and everyone at Community Building Art Works. Poetry can be a life raft in a sea of darkness. I am eternally grateful for your guidance and for helping me find a voice.

To the EMTs, paramedics, and fellow officers of FDNY EMS Station 40 (Sunset Park, Brooklyn): I couldn't ask for a better group of colleagues. The pandemic bent us but we didn't break. I've never been prouder of a group of people than I am of you. A big shout-out to paramedics Stephen (Dr. Strange) Northmore, James (Jimmy Mac) McGuire, Angie (Double A) Alburquerque; to EMTs Kenny (XO) Craig, Juan (Don Juan) Rios, William (Big Bill) Keating, and Alfonso (Bones) Buoninfante, and to all who shared their experiences.

For the dedication and sacrifice of my brothers and sisters in the FDNY EMS, NYC EMS, and in EMS systems everywhere. You are some of the bravest, toughest, and most empathetic people I have ever known. It takes a special kind of someone to become an EMT/paramedic, to step into the unknown, to care for strangers who are sick and injured on a daily basis. A special thank you to my colleagues in AFSCME AFL-CIO DC37, Local 2507, the Uniformed EMTs, Paramedics and Fire Inspectors Union–FDNY; and Local 3621, the Uniformed EMS Officers Union–FDNY. Special thanks to Vincent Variale, president of Local 3621, a mentor who believed in my ability to become the union's vice president.

To my sister-in-law Holly Furio: It's been an interesting journey and I hope for smooth sailing from here on out. To my cousins Walter and Stacy: You are wonderful humans. I cherish the memories of Christmases past and I'm happy life turned out the way it did for you. To my cousins Mimi and Donna, who were there in the early days to share the laughter: I wish you were around to see that you didn't need to live as if there was no tomorrow. To Christopher Chen and Anthony Rivera, my brothers from other mothers: Everywhere I go, you're with me.

In loving memory of all the EMS workers who passed during the pandemic and beyond. Rest in peace—as we say in EMS, we've got it from here.

Among remembrances of those we've lost, I reserve a special place for Greg Hodge, my mentor and friend. These are my people now, Greg. I'll take care of them for you.

And for Cemal (Java Joe) Cengiz: Your death shook me, brother. You will be in my heart forever. I promise to take your advice and slow down.

Someday.

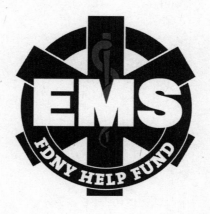

WANT TO MAKE A DIFFERENCE?

Donate to the EMS FDNY Help Fund.

emsfdnyhelpfund.com

WITHDRAWN

6/2022
$26.99